DEDICATION

To Tristan

You are an incredible gift.
Your courage and
bravery inspire me.
The difficulties you face have
made you a deep, compassionate gentleman.
Your father and I are proud of you.

a MOTHER'S GUIDE *to* HERBAL EXTRACTS

a MOTHER'S GUIDE *to* HERBAL EXTRACTS
Saving Tristan

*If the day and night are such
that you greet them with joy
and life emits a fragrance
like flowers
and sweet scented herbs—
that is your success.
All nature is your
congratulations.*

—HENRY DAVID THOREAU

Printed in the United States of America
Second Printing August 2013

Cover design by Kathy Garber

Published by:

The William and Lydia Foundation
P.O. Box 9380
Kalispell, MT 59904
Printed in the United States of America

Author's note:

This book is not intended to replace a one-on-one relationship with a qualified healthcare professional and is not intended as medical advice, but it is a sharing of knowledge and information based on the author's experience.

You are advised and encouraged to consult with your healthcare professional regarding matters concerning your health and, in particular, any symptoms that may require diagnosis or immediate attention.

For more information visit.

www.savingtristan.com

ENDORSEMENTS

Like any of Kathy Garber's unique herbal formulas, Kathy herself is a proprietary blend. The first thing I noticed about her was her modest attire and demeanor. Her soft-spoken Amish culture stood out in the midst of the other clients who came to meet my team at a resort in Mexico. I noticed something else—a fire in her eyes. I was stunned actually. Though quiet, she had that quality of gritty resolve you would expect from a veteran soldier storming the beaches at Normandy in WWII. I soon found out why. She was researching herbs because God had given her a gift, and her son needed a medical miracle. The story of her struggle and her triumph, along with her Amish inventor-husband Nathan, is something you simply MUST read. Together, they heal the sick and have built a business worth millions. I encourage you to stop what you're doing and experience this unusual journey.

—Dr. LANCE WALLNAU | DALLAS, TX

A couple of years ago I confided in a friend that I was having some physical problems. I had gone to a doctor, but I didn't care for the results of the appointment, so I just decided to suffer with it. My friend asked me if I would talk to his friend, Kathy Garber. That meeting changed my life. While I am very thankful for the medical community, I believe that this earth holds the answers to so many of our maladies. Kathy spent time with me and came up with a plan. After one month, I was feeling better than I had in quite a while, and all my symptoms disappeared after a couple of months.

One of my problems was insomnia. As you can imagine, traveling in different time zones throws off your sleeping patterns. Her herbs help no matter what time zone I am in. I can't take melatonin, so this is perfect for me. I travel quite extensively around the world, and while I try to watch what I eat and drink, at times, I drink water and eat foods that are not what I am used to. On one occasion, I felt I had picked up some kind of parasite. I called Kathy and got some of the herbs she recommended. One month later, again, all symptoms were gone. I'm so glad she wrote a book. I'm going to enjoy reading it and implementing it in my life.

—JUDY FRANKLIN | REDDING, CA

I have known and loved the company story and its founding couple, Kathy and Nathan Garber, since I met them in 2005. Working as a team from the beginning, they have maximized their strengths and gifts: Nathan in innovation and sales and Kathy in creating effective herbal formulations from the highest-quality, freshest ingredients. Their teamwork paid off, with thousands benefiting from their efforts as a successful enterprise emerged. I celebrate the cooperation of husband and wife in the creation of something together, and this couple has really excelled in the one-two punch. I think of Kathy every time I take Femme Defense and appreciate her discipline as a scientific technician who has formulated so many herbal combinations for healing. I like the way she combined herbal calcium, enough to meet my need for the day, with other strategic preventative elements and enabled them to flow from a dropper ... brilliant! Our family has enjoyed a large number of products from Mountain Meadow Herbs, and we are so grateful to have this quality source at our fingertips. In fact, whenever we have a peculiar challenge or need support for any physical need, this company has responded with effective custom combinations or, something right off the shelf. They truly understand the interaction of herbs and healing. I give them a 5-Star rating!

—ANNABELLE WALLNAU | DALLAS, TX

When I first started into midwifery seven years ago, I found out that Kathy was making some formulas, so I contacted her as a friend to see whether I could get some through her. I was happy to pass out some of her first catalogs at a midwife meeting and have been using the formulas ever since. God has created herbs for the benefit of mankind, and I'm convinced that the combined use of them complement each other. I'm impressed with the use of these formulas and am thankful for the time and effort that Kathy has put into research and formulating these herbs to meet our needs. I appreciate the response we get when calling Mountain Meadow Herbs with questions and the quick service we get when ordering. May God be glorified as we reach out helping hands to the needs around us!

—ERMA COBLENTZ | CINCINNATI, IA

ACKNOWLEDGEMENTS

I wish to acknowledge and honor those from whose work I have benefited. To the large company of herbalists, researchers, and wise men and women who have labored to discover and share the wonders of natural healing, thank you! Your books have become my mentors and guiding light.

Special thanks to Mark Pederson, author of *Nutritional Herbology*. Your book was my first window of hope for my son, and a decade later, it is still a tattered favorite.

To the many researchers and those who conduct hundreds of thousands of clinical trials and studies around the globe, I am particularly grateful. Your work confirms and illuminates the healing wisdom of less-complicated eras.

I owe much to the creators of *Hyperhealth* software. Thank you for an incredible tool!

To the Mountain Meadow Herbs team, I am forever indebted. You made my dream come true. With unwavering loyalty and dedication, you honored me and my vision beyond what I deserved. You gave me a rare gift, a work community alive with genuine compassion and love. It was an honor to lead you.

To our four beautiful children, Tristan, Brian, Heidi, and Justin, your support and sacrifices are always with me. Thank you for the countless times you cheerfully ate cold dinner because mommy was lost in the world of herbs and forgot to cook.

Lastly, and most importantly, to my husband Nathan, you deserve my lifelong honor and gratitude. Thank you for freeing me to pursue my passion. Without your support and faith in me, I would still live a small life defined by fear. Thank you for laying down your life for me and giving me wings.

—KATHY GARBER

CONTENTS

"God, if You help me figure this out, I will help everyone I can."

I had no idea where these desperate words would lead as they left my lips during the winter of 1996. I was a young twenty-six-year-old mother, broken-hearted by the suffering of my firstborn.

Frequent, painful kidney infections wracked his tiny body in the aftermath of surgery to remove a blockage that had left him with severely damaged kidneys. Dialysis and a kidney transplant in the future were his only hope of survival — not exactly a mother's dream for her child.

I had no idea this unwanted door of suffering would actually open into an exciting world I knew very little about. Finding the courage to push past my son's depressing prognosis was all it took to enter a fascinating realm of discovery, compassion, and destiny.

Although I am a shy, soft-spoken woman with only an eighth-grade formal education, I have been privileged to give our son twelve years of normal life. We have avoided dialysis and transplant largely through the use of natural health solutions, and I have kept my promise: Tens of thousands have benefited from this unusual journey, improving their own health through the herbal formulations I have created with compassion and great care.

—KATHY GARBER

And on the banks of the river,

*there will grow all kinds
of trees for food.*

*Their leaves will not wither,
nor their fruit fail,*

*but they will bear fresh fruit every
month, because the water for
them flows from the sanctuary.*

*Their fruit will be for food,
and their leaves for healing.*

—EZEKIEL 47:12 ESV

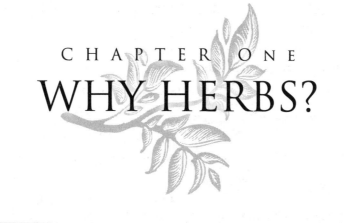

CHAPTER ONE

WHY HERBS?

"My son needs a miracle, or he needs dialysis. There are no other options. Is that right, Dr. Sonnenberg?" I asked with a tremor in my voice.

The kindly doctor's eyes shifted briefly. Then, looking directly into mine, she replied, "Yes, Mrs. Garber, he has about two percent of his kidney function left. He cannot survive much longer without dialysis, and he is too young for a transplant." Again her eyes wandered, this time to our four-year-old son sleeping quietly behind me in the hospital bed. Her voice softened, "I'm sorry. Even if he were my own son, it would be time. We will take him into surgery in the morning." As she walked away, her steps slowed; turning back to me, she added gently, "I have seen a few miracles."

Modern medicine was doing its best to help my firstborn and only child. As I looked into his precious, pale little face, my stomach tightened. Dialysis for the next eight years would drastically change his life, and I questioned his ability to even survive to the required age of twelve for a kidney transplant. We needed a miracle.

In that moment, my father's face came to mind, and I heard again the words I had heard from him so many times, "Kathy, if there is a will, there is a way." I found courage in those simple words on that gray fall day in 1997, courage to seek healing along a path I knew very little about: the wonderful, and what has become to me, the "miracle" world of herbs.

Driven by the need to save my son, studying the use of herbs and nutrition became my new passion. I discovered that plants have been the primary source of healing for centuries, and even today, many drugs are made largely from plant sources. Roots, leaves, bark, flowers, berries, and fruits containing beneficial compounds willingly unfolded their secrets from the pages of fascinating books cluttering our home in the Montana wilderness. Clinical trials and research done at universities were unearthed, giving me hope as they confirmed the ancient wisdom of bygone eras.

Working with our pediatrician, a wonderfully patient doctor whose horizons were open to alternative medicine, I began to apply what I learned. Lab work was done weekly and then monthly as Tristan's kidneys responded to the simple remedies and as toxin levels in his blood began to drop. The adult blood pressure medication was discontinued; he was no longer the pale, anemic child of yesterday.

Active and growing like a weed, he spent his days outside with his BB gun. Rather than being at the dialysis clinic, he was right there to welcome his new little brother in the summer of 1998. His improvement was gradual but amazing, and one year later, when the lab report showed his kidney function to be at ninety percent, being a mom — I cried.

Mom to mom, woman to woman, and friend to friend, I am sharing with you my experience and knowledge in healing with herbs and highly specialized formulations developed through our company, known around the world as Mountain Meadow Herbs. This place is my heart. A brilliantly simple person, I have an unshakable belief in natural healing. I have seen too much success to settle for anything else, and I care too deeply to create anything less than my best.

RESPECT FOR NATURAL HEALING

Dietary supplements are not without controversy, and herbs, in particular, are seen by many as dangerous or risky. Lack of a healthy respect for nature in all its forms is foolhardy and definitely dangerous. None of us can survive without water; however, jumping into the lake during a thunderstorm without knowing how to swim can end the careless person's life. The same is true of herbs: Too much of a good thing in the wrong context can hurt you, but the right herb in the right context can improve and even save a life. Modern medicine undoubtedly saved my son when the blockage responsible for his severe kidney damage was surgically removed when he was two. While I have tremendous respect and gratitude for the advances being made in modern main stream medicine, I cannot ignore the benefits and advantages of nature's gifts or my concern for some aspects of what is now considered "normal" modern medicine.

Drug-related deaths outnumber dietary and herbal-supplement-related deaths by an estimated ratio of 8,000-to-1 in this country. How can 32,000 people die yearly in the United States alone from an adverse reaction to prescription drugs while their preventable, tragic passing goes largely unreported? Could it be because of how common it has become to die from taking a drug that has been approved by the Food and Drug Administration (FDA)? Death by herbs is rare, but it makes a highly unusual story to report on the evening news or daily paper, and it tends to stick in the viewer's mind, creating the illusion that prescription drugs are safer. My instinctive response when asked if herbs are dangerous is, "Dangerous in relation to what? If we are talking herbs as relative to prescription and even over-the-counter (OTC) drugs, then statistically, herbs are clearly the safer option."

Statistics aside, let's look at the Creator's wisdom in just one of nature's offerings. Lobelia is a fascinating plant, valued for its definite antispasmodic, diuretic, and expectorant actions. In Western herbology, it is highly recommended as a balancing herb and as such, is used in many herbal combinations. While classified by some scientists as potentially harmful and its sale banned in Europe, lobelia offers a natural, built-in overdose protection. A punishing round of vomiting awaits those lacking in respect and understanding of its application. Similarly, a remedy that might be perfect for an adult could harm a child, especially one under the age of two. Common sense and the love and care we have for our families should lead to careful, informed decisions in selecting herbal remedies for ourselves and our children.

For me, trying to convince four-year-old Tristan that his survival depended on eating ground-up herbal tablets and powders from capsules mixed with applesauce was a major dilemma. The solution I chose was to substitute less offensive liquid herbal extracts. What I did not know until much later was that I had stumbled across the most effective form of herbal delivery. Those small amber glass bottles with rubber-topped droppers held the precious liquid extracts of herbs that gave my son a normal life, and in this form, he didn't mind taking his medicine at all! Known as tinctures or extracts, these powerful liquids are up to 70 percent more effective than tablets or encapsulated herbs. According to Terry Willard, Ph.D. of the Wild Rose College and author of the textbook Modern Herbology, this improvement is due to the liquid form being more easily assimilated into the body and the alcohol acting as an effective carrier into the blood stream. This benefit is particularly valuable when the patient needs quick relief or is in an acute situation.

Herbal extracts or tinctures are liquids created when the beneficial properties of the herb have been pulled out of the plant using a liquid extracting medium. Alcohol, water, glycerin, and even vinegar are used as mediums. A mixture of alcohol and water are the most common choice. Widely available both online and in health food stores, these herbal extracts and tinctures are often overlooked by those in search of natural healing. When ordering these products, always choose a reputable brand, and if you do not experience improvement, try another label. My first purchases were from WishGarden Herbs, a small company in Oregon, and I was very happy with their products.

As Tristan's health continued to improve, my confidence in natural healing grew. In 2001, I began making my own golden, liquid extracts from various herbs and combining them to meet my son's need for highly specialized formulations. I chose to use as small an amount of alcohol as possible, and I used distilled water and glycerin as the main extracting medium. Creating, with my own hands, the means of survival for our son was vastly empowering, and my heart was repeatedly overcome with gratitude as I prepared these remedies from natural, God-given sources.

As Tristan's health continued to improve, my confidence in natural healing grew.

Herbal remedies are beautiful in that, unlike drugs, they are less expensive and they rarely have side effects. For example, because insomnia is a problem for hundreds of thousands of Americans, drug companies cash in on the need for sleep to the tune of $1.3 billion annually (just on the two most popular drugs alone). If you have ever used an OTC medication or prescription drug to help you sleep, you no doubt, are familiar with the usual next-day grogginess, depression, and headaches. Perhaps you have also worried about all those, frightening, possibly serious side effects listed on the printout that was handed to you by your pharmacist or listed in small print on the product packaging. Herbs such as Valerian Root, Hops Flowers, Scullcap, and Passionflower can help you fall asleep and stay asleep without any side effects, especially when taken in a liquid combination.

The dreaded side effects accompanying the adult blood pressure medication, which my son originally needed to lower his out-of-control blood pressure, were very motivating as I studied and researched for better options. After two weeks of applying what I was learning, Tristan's blood pressure returned to normal and has been within the normal range ever since. The herbs I selected, along with Coenzyme Q10, were doing more for him than the prescription drug had been able to accomplish. He no longer needed help walking, and the dizziness and nausea, side effects of the blood pressure medicine, also vanished, allowing him to enjoy a full life, as all little boys should.

The dollars spent over the past twelve years to give Tristan a normal life through natural treatment have been a mere fraction of what would have been the cost of eight years of dialysis followed by a risky kidney transplant. In the United States, healthcare represents a sixth of our nation's economy, and costs continue to rise. The fierce battle in Washington, along with the outcry from the people, is evidence of how important and even emotional this issue is to all of us. Vicious arguments focus on money, extending coverage to those who cannot afford healthcare, forcing unwilling participants to participate in government programming, and finding the funds to pay for new programs.

To those who are sickened by the whole mess and who believe in taking personal responsibility for their own health, natural healing presents an amazing alternative. Many herbal remedies and dietary supplements have now been scientifically proven to restore health and help prevent diseases otherwise requiring high-dollar treatment. The information is out there, and if this book is the beginning of your own quest for answers for you or your loved ones, congratulations! I hope you will continue your search and find your solution regardless of any disadvantages you face. As a young, inexperienced mom, I found my own desperately needed answers without the benefit of education beyond high school.

Courage and determination, bolstered by prayer and faith, were enough for me and can be for you too.

SPECIAL NOTE

My journey into the world of herbal medicine has been long and detailed. From years of research, study, and experimentation, I have created effective herbal combinations to address specific conditions and general health concerns. For the readers' benefit, these original formulations will appear in bold print throughout this book and are available from stores listed at **www.savingtristan.com** *and from Mountain Meadow Herbs.*

CHAPTER TWO
HERBS MADE EASY

This is the information age. In all of history, there has never been so much valuable and even life-saving information at our fingertips. Today, a software program containing all the information found in a room full of books can be bought. Libraries are a great resource for anyone wanting to explore the wonderful world of herbs. Clinical trials and ongoing research can be followed online. Many community colleges offer courses in herbal medicine and natural wellness. Since books have always been a passion of mine, naturally, I turned to books. A kind friend who was studying to become a master herbalist lent me her textbooks, which I devoured.

Hyperhealth software is a spectacular resource that every mom with a computer should own. It is very easy to use. Enter any condition into the index, and instantly see a list of all herbs, dietary supplements, and even foods that can be used to address this particular condition. Both information on clinical trials and any research done on the suggested herbs are given as well. A word of caution, it is easy to spend a lot more time discovering and learning than intended!

Walking to the well-stocked, herbal remedy cupboard and choosing a bottle with confidence is so much easier for the educated and prepared mom than an expensive and even potentially hazardous trip to the doctor's office. Johnny and his siblings are exposed to all kinds of germs and diseases just from time spent sitting together in the waiting room. Chances are your call for an appointment was met with "I'm sorry, but Dr. Jones is not able to see Johnny today. He is completely booked. You can bring him into our walk-in clinic where he will be seen as soon as possible."

Those words are enough to make a caring mom cry, knowing her child will not receive the attention he deserves. After hours of waiting to be seen by a complete stranger, there is the trip to the pharmacy and another wait. Half a day later, you are finally home with a headache, struggling to get the drug you're not sure about into the screaming child. Brother is grumpy and upset because lunch is late and it's nap time. Sound familiar? What if it were possible to avoid this fiasco and have your sick child rest and recover at home because you are prepared and know how to take care of an earache without an antibiotic?

CONSISTENCY IS THE KEY

Preventing illness by strengthening the immune system with herbs can make those dreaded trips to the doctor's office after a sleepless night a rare occurrence. Consistency is the key to addressing chronic conditions such as recurrent respiratory infections, joint problems, issues resulting from stress, and nutritive support regimens such as calcium supplements. Dosing one to three times a day, before or between meals is a great pattern to follow for three to six months. Nutritive supplements such as calcium should be taken on an ongoing basis.

Timing in taking herbal extracts is also determined by the benefit you seek. For example, if you need help falling asleep, drink a relaxing cup of tea thirty minutes before bedtime. Since it takes five to fifteen minutes for the herbs in liquid form to enter the system, take a combination of herbal extracts containing Valerian, Hops and Passionflower soon after finishing the tea. Prepare for bed, and if you are still awake ten minutes later, take an additional dose. Repeat if necessary. The same procedure can be used for relieving menstrual cramps, growing pains, and headaches.

The value of being well-prepared for when illness hits cannot be over stressed. Herbal remedies tend to work best at the onset of illness, before the viral or bacterial invasion has gathered strength and increased in numbers. If a rushed trip has to be made to the health food store for the needed remedy, assuming the store is open, valuable time is lost and anxiety will cloud your mind at a time when it needs to be at its best. The

The value of being well-prepared when illness hits cannot be over stressed.

wise mother will not rely only on herbal remedies during illness. Vitamins A, C, and E, along with glyconutrients, good hydration, and plenty of rest are all important for a safe and rapid recovery.

The frequency of taking extracts changes during illness. Most can be taken every two hours while the condition is peaking in intensity and even every 30 minutes, in some cases. Begin taking the herbal remedies and repeat every two hours for 12 hours as soon as symptoms of illness such as cold, flu, urinary tract, or respiratory infections appear. Often the illness is stopped in its tracks, particularly for those whose diet is rich in fruits and vegetables and low in sugar. On the other hand, the lack of fresh air, sunshine, and exercise cannot be corrected simply by taking dietary supplements.

Putting an herbal extract directly under the tongue and holding it there is the fastest way to get herbs into the system. However, this is rarely necessary, and most tinctures don't taste that great. Diluting the herbal extract in a bit of warm water or juice is preferred by most people. Orange juice is especially effective in masking the more bitter herbs such as Gentian, which is used to rid the body of parasites. Children are much more willing to take this type of treatment when the unpleasant flavor is masked in something they enjoy. Glycerites and the extracts of non-bitter herbs made with organic grain alcohol taste more pleasant and are easy to take directly.

Body weight is important to consider in determining the appropriate dosage for adults and children. In general 1/4 to 1/2 teaspoon is used by adults weighing 120–150 pounds. Since most extracts come in glass bottles with rubber topped droppers, it is easy to simply use the dropper, which will contain approximately 1/8 teaspoon, to measure dosage. This is the amount that is easily drawn into the pipette by squeezing the bulb. It will not be full. If you buy extracts in different sizes, check the amount the dropper holds with a measuring spoon. To determine the dosage for a child follow Clark's Rule.

CLARK'S RULE

Divide the child's weight in pounds by 150 to get the approximate fraction of the adult dose to give to the child.

Example: For a 30-pound child, give 1/5 (or 30/150) of the adult's dose. So, if the adult dose is 1/4 teaspoon, or two droppers, taken 3 times a day, the child's dose will be a little less than 1/2 dropper, still taken 3 times a day.

Be prepared to observe your child carefully as you begin using herbal extracts. Some children are much more sensitive and will respond very quickly to small amounts. Others may need slightly more of the same herb and for a longer period of time to get the same response. Infants should be carefully observed for 15 to 20 minutes after first giving an herbal extract to make sure there is no unwanted reaction such as a skin outbreak or any change in breathing.

Since only the most benign herbs are appropriate for infants, an allergic reaction is highly unlikely, but until you have tested and know your baby's response, take the time to make sure that all is well. Your confidence will grow with experience. Enjoy the learning process. While there is no end to discovery in the amazing realm of natural healing with herbs, you only need enough information to solve the issues affecting you and your family, and that knowledge is well within your reach.

CHAPTER THREE
HERBS FOR THE NEW AND EXPECTING MOM

Herbs can support the new and expectant mom by providing part of the additional nourishment needed and by easing many of the discomforts experienced during pregnancy, childbirth, and the nursing period. As caring mothers, the safety of our unborn or nursing child is foremost in our minds, and everything that passes our lips undergoes the test, "Will this hurt my baby?"

While many herbs have been safely and successfully used during pregnancy and while nursing, it is important to consider the safety of any herbal product during this time. All herbs with a laxative effect should be avoided. Other commonly used herbs to avoid are **Feverfew, Uva Ursi,** and **Golden Seal.** When in doubt, always check with your midwife or healthcare provider or refer to a good herbal text. Resist the idea that every product is safe just because it is natural or herbal. Pregnancy and new motherhood are beautiful times. They are your opportunity to partner with God in the miracle of life, and in this helpful chapter, you will discover God-given plants and nutrients to make being a mom a little easier.

HERBAL CALCIUM

First, calcium is your best friend, especially when taken daily in a liquid combination extracted from herbs rich in calcium and magnesium. Your body will thank you. The old saying "a tooth is lost with each child carried and birthed" is accurate for many women who fail to provide the extra calcium the body needs as their little one develops. Aching joints, nervousness, fatigue, leg cramps, and tooth decay can all be signs your body is begging for more calcium.

Among the herbs highest in calcium is a prickly little plant known as **Stinging Nettle.** Most hikers are familiar with its stinging burn. Not a loner, calcium needs magnesium, a calcium carrier, to transport it in and out of the cell membranes for effective delivery and absorption. **Oat Straw** ranked best in a study done by research chemist Mark Pederson on magnesium sources. **Horsetail** is unique among herbs containing silicon in a bioavailable form. Silicon assists calcium in the maintenance and growth of bones, joints, and collagen levels. **Corn Silk** is widely used to soothe irritated bladder tissue, to prevent bedwetting, and is rich in calcium. Perhaps the best-known herb, **Chamomile,** is well studied and often included in skeletal combinations because of its smooth muscle relaxing and anti-inflammatory properties. **Scullcap** adds a calming, anti-spasmodic effect and helps you get a well-deserved, good night's rest. This combination of herbs, **Herbal Calcium,** is my personal favorite of all the formulations I have created.

Lack of calcium, accompanied by too little rest, can play a major role in not having enough milk to satisfy your baby. Today, doctors who used to recommend formula are encouraging new mothers to give their baby the best diet: mom's milk. Studies show that the benefits of nursing your child extend beyond the toddler days into adulthood. Nursing a baby when all goes well is like a satisfying dream. You are at peace knowing your baby is getting the best nourishment possible. There is no impatient screaming from a hungry baby waiting for the formula to be mixed or for bottles to be washed and sterilized. Nursing is healthy, cost-effective, easy, and convenient. However, it is common for committed nursing moms to face feeding challenges, and meeting the demands of a rapidly growing infant can be frustrating to say the least.

Factors contributing to not having enough milk vary. However, there are wonderful herbs available to both increase and enrich milk production. For example, if Prolactin, an important hormone that regulates milk supply and is controlled by the pituitary gland, is not doing its job, **Chaste Berry** is nature's amazing answer. It can correct any existing imbalance by regulating prolactin release. **Stinging Nettle, Alfalfa, Red Raspberry,** and **Blessed Thistle** are used to enrich breast milk. **Anise Seed, Milk Thistle** and **Fennel Seed** stimulate and increase milk production.

Anxiety about the ability to nurse, along with the stress of caring for a new baby, can also keep your body from producing enough milk. **Lemon Balm** and **Scullcap** are relaxing and calming, while **Peppermint** is soothing to both mother and child. Sore nipples are enough to cause even the most committed mother to reconsider her decision to breastfeed. Thankfully, **Marshmallow Root** is soothing to irritated tissue, particularly the skin and mucous membranes. Candida is the culprit in some cases, but **Scullcap** can be helpful in normalizing the overgrowth and preventing thrush. **Maxi-Milk,** is a combination of these herbs in liquid extract form. Based on customer feedback, more milk can be expected as early as within twenty-four hours after taking the first dose.

Midwives have used and promoted herbal remedies for many years to tone and prepare the body for giving birth. For most women, giving birth naturally and painlessly has yet to be discovered. However, there are herbs whose effects on the uterus and the systems involved in childbirth are very valuable. **Red Raspberry Leaf** is the most popular uterine tonic and enjoys an excellent reputation as the single most important herb to prepare a woman's body for giving birth and to reduce the pain of childbirth.

Wild Yam and **Squawvine** can gently relieve anxiety, late-pregnancy discomfort, and excessive pain during birth. The bitter compounds in **False Unicorn** have a normalizing and enhancing effect on the uterus and ovaries and can be helpful for moms who tend to carry past their due date or have long labors. **Blue Cohosh** is widely used to bring on effective contractions, so it should be taken with caution during late pregnancy or as part of an herbal combination. **Blessed Thistle, Scullcap, Motherwort**, and **Ginger** can be used as late-pregnancy tonics because of their calming, soothing effect. A small amount of **Bayberry** may help prevent excessive bleeding.

At the request of my mother-in-law, a midwife for 26 years, I created a combination of these herbal extracts from an old manual, adjusted it based on more modern studies, and named it **Gentle Birth Formula**. Responses from grateful new moms poured in and confirmed that birth can indeed be a gentle, natural process. On a personal note, I used this combination in preparation for giving birth to our last two children. Previous labors had been long and very difficult — 28 and 17 hours of blood, sweat, and tears. With the help of herbs, our daughter was in my arms after six hours of labor, and our third son entered the world after four short hours. There is no question as to which labor I preferred!

AFTER THE BABY IS BORN

After-pains can block the joy of holding your precious new daughter or son, herbs are a wonderful gift at this time. **Crampbark** and **Black Haw** have an almost immediate and direct effect on the uterus, especially in liquid extract form. They are among the best remedies for quickly relieving after-pains. **St. John's Wort** and **Yarrow** are also helpful. Nursing can also bring on after-pains during the first few weeks, but keeping a bottle of **After-Pain Relief** within easy reach and repeating the dosage until the pain lessens is safe and appropriate.

Your body goes through intense changes during pregnancy and especially during childbirth. Hormone levels do not always return to normal on their own and can leave a new mom feeling unexplainably sad, with thoughts and emotions not normally experienced. This is often referred to as the "baby blues." Herbs such as **Chaste Berry, False Unicorn,** and **Sarsaparilla** have a balancing effect on hormone levels. Adding female tonics such as **Blessed Thistle** and **Squawvine** along with the harmonizing effect of **Licorice** and **Ginger** can make a world of difference. **HB Formula** is combination of these herbs.Postpartum depression is more serious, and caution should be used in addressing it with herbs.

STOMACH AID FOR NAUSEA

For the woman who is suffering the nausea known as "morning sickness," **Ginger** is your new best friend! A combination of fresh and dried **Ginger** extract was shown to eliminate or reduce nausea and vomiting in eighty percent of the women suffering from morning sickness who participated in a clinical trial. Digestion slows as high levels of estrogen circulate. **Peppermint** and **Fennel** counteract this by stimulating digestion and preventing uncomfortable gas from forming.

If you have a history of morning sickness, doing a liver and whole body cleanse before conceiving may help. Such preventative treatment has helped other women avoid this miserable experience. **Liver Glow II** contains **Lemon Balm, Alfalfa, Milk Thistle, Dandelion, Grape Seed,** and **Olive Leaf.** This combination safely supports your liver during pregnancy and may be all you need to feel better. These herbs can be taken with **Stomach Aid.** Herbal support of the liver can also help relieve the exhaustion so many moms experience while expecting because both the liver and the adrenal glands are responsible for meeting most of our energy needs.

Located at the top of the kidneys, the adrenal glands increase in size and activity during pregnancy. They are responsible for producing hormones that respond to stress and affect blood pressure and blood sugar levels. **Astragalus**, **Rhodiola**, **Eleuthero,** and **Wild Yam** are all wonderful supports for the adrenal glands in their important roles. **Adren-L-Aid II**

STRENGTHENING WITH HERBAL IRON

Anemia also can cause fatigue, but iron-rich foods such as red meat can be very unappealing during pregnancy. Instead of increasing hemoglobin with ferrous sulfate, **Stinging Nettle**, **Dandelion Root,** and **Yellow Dock** make an excellent alternative. This combination is popular among midwives. Originally, it was created for my mother-in-law who saw low hemoglobin levels rise in a matter of weeks.

High blood pressure during pregnancy can become a serious complication, especially for the five percent of women who develop toxemia. Calcium, magnesium, and selenium have been studied as preventatives and have offered positive outcomes. **Herbal Calcium,** mentioned at the beginning of this chapter, is rich in these nutrients. In general, **Herbal Calcium** is safe during pregnancy. The beginning of your second trimester is a good time to start taking it. When a history of toxemia is present or blood pressure is elevated, **Herbal Calcium** can be taken during the first trimester.

Coenzyme Q10 has an amazing effect on the cardiovascular system and kidneys. When buying Coenzyme Q10, be sure to choose an oil-base gel cap. Dry powder in a capsule has been shown to be much less effective. **Gingko Biloba** and **Hawthorn** improve heart function and lower blood pressure by dilating blood vessels. **Bilberry** and **Ginger** improve blood circulation. **Herbal CardioCare** is a combination of these herbs and can generally be safely used during pregnancy. The dosage can be repeated as needed, within reason, when there is a need to lower blood pressure quickly. Drinking five cups of decaffeinated green tea daily can also be beneficial. Full benefit of these herbs and supplements can take up to two weeks to be realized, so be patient.

Full benefit of herbs and supplements take time to be realized, so be patient.

Bulging varicose veins are not only unsightly, but they can also be very painful. In 2004, I received a note from a customer who loved the **Gentle Birth Formula** and wanted to know if she could take it throughout her next pregnancy since the pain from her varicose veins disappeared during the five weeks she had used it. I was intrigued, and since the Gentle Birth Formula is designed only for the final weeks before giving birth, I mailed her a combination of **Bilberry Leaf, Bilberry, and Bayberry,** as they are known to strengthen the capillaries, prevent abnormal blood clotting, and relieve the pain associated with varicose veins. She soon let me and her midwife know that the results were outstanding, and soon, orders came in for what is now known as **Vari-Plex.**

Additionally, herbal lotions that soothe, cool, and tighten are available. Kettle Care makes an excellent one with all organic ingredients and sold as **Vascular Ease Lotion.** Carrying a baby for nine months does not have to necessitate enduring the pain, itching, and burning of varicose veins.

Approximately 20 percent, or one of every five pregnancies, ends in loss. Of that number, most miscarriages occur within the first 12 weeks. There may be a genetic disorder or a problem with mom, dad, or the baby; and often there is no answer or explanation at all. Using a combination of herbs to calm the uterus, relieve stress, and balance hormones can be helpful. Inevitable miscarriage (one in which the baby has died) is not prolonged by using these herbs. **Black Haw** is used by European physicians and modern herbalists to calm and relax the uterus. **Cramp Bark** relieves cramping and pain and calms the nerves. **False Unicorn** has a balancing effect on female hormones. **Wild Yam** is traditionally used to ease muscle spasms and to stimulate the adrenal glands. Anxiety can be gently relieved by **Passion Flower,** which calms the nerves and promotes restful sleep. **C&B Formula** is a combination of these herbs, 1/2 teaspoon can be taken every 2–3 hours until the cramping and bleeding lessens, followed by 1/4 teaspoon one to three times daily as needed.

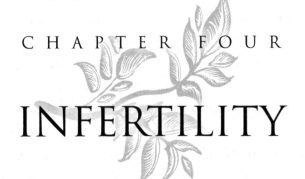

CHAPTER FOUR

INFERTILITY

"Mrs. Garber, you have secondary infertility. Both of your tubes are completely blocked, and you have endometriosis. It is highly unlikely you will ever conceive again." Suddenly, I was shocked to discover I had joined two million women whose dreams of a family are crushed annually in our country. I was still young and healthy, and having grown up with six siblings, I desperately wanted more than one child. Since the medical world offered little hope, I turned to my faith and did a daring thing.

I asked God to tell me if there would be more children, but I also told Him I would always love and serve Him regardless of the answer. I just needed to know.

In my heart, I heard a gentle whisper, "You will be the mother of children." Eight years later to that very day, I found myself holding the newborn we had fought and believed for, our beautiful and only daughter Heidi. With her tiny wet fingers gripping one of mine, I cried and gave thanks for another miracle.

Many factors contribute to the inability to conceive. The problem can be traced to either partner. Endometriosis, scar tissue from C-sections, hormone imbalance, yeast overgrowth, toxic overload, smoking, and other habits detrimental to optimal health can all play a part. Be prepared to be patient if you wish to increase your fertility through natural means. I have had the great pleasure and honor of helping many women uncover the source of their problem and go on to become mothers. In some instances, it happened as quickly as a few weeks, while for others it took up to two years.

Creating and providing natural solutions to relieve suffering is always rewarding. I keep a special file filled with birth announcements and letters from women I have been honored to help. It is one of my most precious treasures. Herbs are a wonderful alternative to the painful, invasive, and often ineffective methods used by modern medicine. For many would-be parents, the cost alone is frightening and often is not covered by insurance. Simple life style changes, prayer, and dietary supplements are all within reach.

Before you stimulate your body with herbs and supplements to enhance fertility, it is wise to cleanse it and your lifestyle as well. You may discover that all your body needed was relief from a toxic overload caused by the many chemicals in your environment, the food you eat, and the habits you have accepted such as consuming caffeine, tobacco, and alcohol. In my experience, three months of cleansing the entire body, paying close attention to cleansing, and supporting any particular organ that shows signs of being in need has helped many women go on to become mothers after struggling with years of infertility. Rated number one by *Natural Health* magazine, the **Whole Body/Colon Cleanse** from the Pure Body Institute is my favorite as an excellent and affordable cleanse.

Endometriosis is considered the leading cause of infertility in women. It causes painful periods and heavy bleeding as the lining of the uterus grows outside its normal boundaries. Reaching into the fallopian tubes, endometriosis can block the meeting of the egg and sperm and interfere with normal conception. A combination of toning, balancing, and cleansing herbs such as those found in the **T&C Formula** can do wonders in relieving the pain and normalizing estrogen levels, which are thought to contribute to endometriosis. **Yarrow** and **Chamomile** are used to clear congestion and soothe inflammation of the female organs. **Red Raspberry, Blue Cohosh**, **Licorice**, and **Mistletoe** are excellent uterine tonics, **Dong Quai** and **Red Raspberry** decrease heavy menstrual flow without stopping it. Pain can be eased by adding **Ginger** and **Capsicum,** while **False Unicorn** reduces swelling and inflammation and normalizes estrogen levels.

The mutation of candida into a fungal infection, or what is commonly known as a yeast infection, is another burden to rid the body of when preparing to conceive. **Pau D'Arco Bark, Licorice, Chamomile, Barberry,** and **Oregon Grape Root** control the proliferation of candida and fight fungal infections. **Gotu Kola's** saponins have a weakening effect on membranous tissue, making it easier for the above herbs to do their work. **Cat's Claw** cleanses and reduces inflammation in the entire gastrointestinal tract, while **Marshmallow** soothes irritation. **Ginger** neutralizes toxins, while **Sarsaparilla** binds the endotoxins that gain entry into the blood stream and facilitates their elimination from the body.

Since yeast infections are often difficult to eliminate, it is important to use herbal remedies for at least three months. It is also necessary for both partners to participate in the cleansing process. Alternating two effective combinations such as **Yeast X I** and **Yeast X II** every two weeks can prevent the build-up of immunity to the herbs. Because die-off can cause headaches, nausea, and increased itching, include **probiotics** and **Sarsaparilla** to keep the process more comfortable. Avoid white flour, sugary foods, and drinks. Instead, focus on vegetables, nuts, and whole foods.

Parasites are another unnecessary burden that can easily be addressed with herbs. **Green Black Walnut Hull** extract, **Wormwood,** and **Cloves** are powerful anti- parasitical herbs. They should be added during the second month of cleansing with the **Whole Body/Colon Cleanse**. Be sure they are including in any parasite cleanse you choose. Researcher Dr. Hulda Clark makes a convincing connection between infertility and parasites in her book, *The Cure for All Diseases*. Among her findings is the presence of the flatworm in every case of endometriosis. Due to the proximity of the anus to the vagina, it is easy for parasites to take up residence within the female organs. Don't skip this important step for both partners in preparing to conceive. For more information on herbs and parasites, see Chapter Five.

HB FORMULA FOR HORMONE IMBALANCE

Irregularity or absence of periods also contributes to infertility. If you have never had a period, it is important to see a doctor to confirm that all female organs are present. While such a condition is rare, for your own peace of mind, have a doctor rule it out. If all is well, you will be more confident in the next steps. Hormone imbalance may be the cause of both irregular and absent cycles. In various studies, **Chaste Tree Berry** has been found to be effective in normalizing Follicle-Stimulating Hormone (FSH) levels, lowering elevated estrogen levels, stimulating the production of progesterone, and normalizing the production and secretion of the luteinizing hormone. Here again, **False Unicorn** is valuable in helping to bring on and regulate periods. When combined with other female tonics and stimulants such as **Sarsaparilla, Blessed Thistle**, **Squawvine,** and **Ginger,** irregular cycles can be corrected.

Natural progesterone cream can bring on a period and regulate an irregular cycle. In the absence of a normal cycle, use as directed for 45 days, and then discontinue. Your period should begin within a day or two. If your cycles are irregular, apply the cream from day 12 through day 26, with day one being the first day of your period. Select a progesterone cream made from **Mexican Wild Yam** and packaged in an air-tight container. One with a pump will also save you the hassle of measuring.

If you are young and enjoy excellent health, your body may simply need the stimulation found in supplements traditionally used to increase fertility, some of which are now backed by scientific research. In a clinical trial, **Chaste Tree Berry** was found to increase fertility in eighty percent of women between the ages of 23 and 36. **Dong Quai** is the herb of choice among naturopaths and herbalists in addressing infertility. **False Unicorn,** with its balancing effect on the female hormones, is an obvious choice as well. **Eleuthero** can minimize any negative effect that stress may have on fertility.

In the early days of studying herbs and creating formulations, I received a call from a family member struggling with infertility. I created a combination of the herbs discussed in the previous paragraph and mailed it to her. I was pleasantly shocked to receive another call six weeks later announcing a positive pregnancy test! Today, she and many others are enjoying the gift of a child through simple God-given gifts that are found in nature instead of at the local fertility clinic. In honor of the promise given to women by the Creator, this formula is known as **Fruitful Vine**.

Vitamin C is an extremely important supplement for increasing fertility naturally. Studies indicate that progesterone levels increase significantly. In one study, the author found treatment with Vitamin C alone resulted in the commencement of ovulation in 40 percent of the subjects, with 21 percent conceiving during the six months of treatment. Up to 10,000 mgs can be taken safely on a daily basis. Select a Vitamin C made from plant food sources rather than one from a synthetic form. Discontinue large doses as soon as pregnancy is confirmed. As an additional precaution, it is wise not to exceed 2,000 mgs per day after ovulation (mid-cycle) to reduce the risk of miscarriage.

JUST FOR MEN: LEGA-C-HERBS AND PROGENTOR VI

Infertility is not just a woman's problem, but nature has answers for men as well. Cleansing the whole body is a good place to start, especially paying attention to any organ showing signs of stress or disease. Many men seldom receive the essential vitamins and minerals pertinent to their reproductive health. Choose a multivitamin carefully insuring that it contains **Zinc** and **Selenium** to enhance sperm production and motility, and vitamins **A, C, E, B12,** and **Folic Acid** to increase sperm count and quality. In studies, **Coenzyme Q10** was shown to energize sperm. Avoid wearing tight-fitting under garments or trousers and sitting in hot tubs for prolonged periods.

The herb **Tribulus Terrestris** has become very popular among men in recent years. It is helpful in stimulating sperm production, increasing sperm survival time, and producing seminal fluid. The antioxidant properties of **Astragulus** and **Eleuthero** may protect and maintain sperm cells and increase their motility. **Pygeum** may improve the quality of seminal fluid, **Barrenwort,** formerly known as Horny Goat Weed, is used to increase seminal fluid and to relieve impotence or the inability to maintain erection. **Yohimbe, Ginkgo Biloba, Ashwaganda, Eleuthero,** and **Tribulus Terrestris** can improve normal male responsiveness.

Simply understanding your cycles and being able to clearly identify the signals your body is sending during ovulation can make the difference between being childless and enjoying a newborn. *Taking Charge of Your Fertility,* by Toni Welcher, is the best resource I have found on this subject. The book is easy to read and thoroughly explains the Fertility Awareness Method, which, in a few minutes a day, allows you to maximize your chance of conception. This resource has helped hundreds of thousands of women conceive, avoid conception naturally, or simply gain a better understanding of how their amazing reproductive system works.

Knowing where to begin to naturally improve your fertility does not need to be intimidating. If both partners are generally in good health, start with a **whole body/colon cleanse** for three months, and include a parasite cleanse. If you have not yet had any testing done to determine where the problem lies, you can choose the less-expensive route of trying herbs to stimulate fertility in both of you before you see a doctor and have costly tests done. Cleansing and educating yourself to identify the signs of ovulation are your next steps.

For those who are in poor health and have various complaints, begin with a **whole body/colon cleanse** for three months and a parasite cleanse. If you suspect yeast infection or endometriosis or you have ovarian cysts or irregular cycles, address these next in the order of what is causing you the most discomfort. Build up any organ you suspect to be weak, such as the liver or the kidneys. Glands, including the thyroid and the adrenals, should also be supported in your effort to become healthy enough to conceive and carry the baby to full term. This attention to your body may be all you need. If it is not, now you can clearly recognize the signs of ovulation, and the next step is to start taking the right herbs to increase fertility.

CHAPTER FIVE

ORGAN CLEANSING, PARASITES, AND YEAST INFECTIONS

I magine living in your home for 20 years and never cleaning it. The buildup of dirt and clutter would make it an unpleasant and unhealthy place to be. While we wash our cars and we insist on gleaming floors and sparkling windows, we tend to give little thought to cleansing our organs. Environmental toxins build up and eliminative channels become sluggish and clogged. New chemicals find their way into our food supply every year, and we wonder why we feel so poorly. Growing numbers of leading researchers and health professionals believe that thoroughly cleansing the body is the number one method of health improvement.

Cleansing has gained popularity in recent years, and today, there is an astonishing and bewildering array of cleanses available. Some focus on one organ, such as the liver; others promise a new life through a clean colon. Some are gentle, but others are so intense that you cannot leave the house for fear of urgently needing a restroom. Liquid cleanses in giant bottles, powders to be mixed with water or juice, and cleansing teas all, no doubt, contain wonderful cleansing compounds, but my experience has been that, in general, they taste awful. So in my case, in spite of my best intentions, after a few days, the thought of downing a big glass of slimy, gritty, or bitter liquid was too much, and the full benefit of the cleanse was never realized.

In searching for a cleansing product that I could offer our clients with confidence, I discovered a gentle but effective one made by the Pure Body Institute. Designed to cleanse all the major organs, it can be bought with or without the Colon Cleanse. This remedy perfectly suits my idea of what a cleanse should be and is easy to take in pill form for the suggested three months. While you will notice increased elimination, you can continue your daily routine without fear. Many doctors are recommending this excellent cleanse and offer presentations to learn more about its benefits. This is a good place to start for anyone interested in cleansing the body, and for best results, do take it for the suggested three months, once or twice a year.

PARASITES

Parasitic worms travel through the blood stream and can invade any organ. As all your organs are being cleansed, stimulated, and unclogged, this is an important issue to address **during the second month of cleansing**. We would all like to think we and our families are free of these silent invaders who survive on the nutrients meant for us and cause a myriad of symptoms and diseases. The reality is that up to eighty percent of us are hosts. Their eggs find their way into our bodies through direct human contact, contaminated food and water, farm animals, household pets, and undercooked meats. More than 100 types of parasite worms can live happily in human bodies.

The work of the late researcher Dr. Hulda Clark is perhaps the most important in making the connection between parasites and disease. Her fascinating book, *The Cure for All Diseases* is a valuable, easy-to-read resource on this subject. Symptoms of parasites range from annoying to life threatening and can include any or all of the following:

- itching nose and anus
- chronic constipation
- frequent gas and bloating
- skin irritations and rashes
- eczema
- loss of appetite
- whip worm
- headaches
- abdominal pain
- failure to thrive in children
- insomnia
- irritability
- mental dullness
- dry skin and hair
- excess weight
- weight loss
- asthma
- dizziness

- vomiting
- gallstones
- endometriosis
- food and soil cravings

Wormwood, Cloves, and **Green Black Walnut Hull** extract are powerful anti-parasiticals and should be included in the parasite cleanse you choose. **Green Tea** extract is a powerful antioxidant and increases the effect of **Wormwood. Quassia** also destroys parasites and, as a bitter tonic, improves the appetite. **Gentian** and **Elecampane** root tone and soothe the digestive tract and lower bowel transit time. Elecampane is also anti-parasitical, **Fennel** seed extract is interesting in that one researcher found it has the ability to intoxicate worms. In their inebriated state, they leave their homes and are eliminated.

The herbs in the previous paragraph are all powerful and part of the **Para-Rid** formula. I added **Ginger, Catnip,** and **Fennel** to ease stomach cramps caused by gas or griping, creating a very child-friendly parasite cleanse. In liquid extract form, it is easy to add **Para-Rid** to an acidic juice such as orange, tomato or grape to mask the worst of the bitterness. Caution should be used in ridding children who are under two years of age of parasites. **Olive leaf** extract is an appropriate option, but do observe your child carefully for gums that swell or bleed, and lower the dosage if needed.

Born of the desperation to resolve our youngest son's severe eczema and nighttime coughing, I broke the rules and gave him five drops each of **Para-Rid** and **Clark FX** (a combination of **Green Black Walnut Hull** extract, **Wormwood,** and **Cloves**) at the age of 18 months. He was not responding to the Olive leaf extract. After three days of this small dosage three times each day, the coughing stopped and never returned. His skin condition improved dramatically, and within a few weeks, he only had a small area on the back of one knee. If you find it necessary to use the stronger herbs for a child under two, be very careful. Offer small dosages for short periods of time only.

Roundworm, or the ascaris, is so common in adults and children that as many as a hundred million people may be infected worldwide. Causing asthma, rashes, abdominal pain, appetite loss, and intestinal blockages, this parasite grows up to 12 inches long and can lay 200,000 eggs per day. In addition to herbs, **Coenzyme Q10** is helpful in cleansing the body of roundworms and tapeworms. Since they are larger worms with many eggs inside, it is important to do the full six-day treatment two times. If your symptoms persist, see *The Cure for All Diseases* for ozonated olive oil and zapping. Be sure to cleanse any yeast infection as well. Parasites live in and are further carried through the body by detrimental yeast cells.

Roundworm may infect as many as a hundred million people worldwide.

The timing of taking herbs to rid your body of parasites is also important. Worms, like fish, lay their eggs around the time of the full moon, so begin treatment two days before full moon for a total of six days or as directed on the cleanse you choose.

Repeat the following month beginning again two days before full moon. As preventive maintenance, **Para-Rid** or **Clark FX** can be used one day a week. This regimen is particularly helpful if you live on a farm or have pets. Include your pets in the treatment as well. Foreign travel certainly calls for a parasite cleanse on return, or better yet, if the visit is short, take the herbs with you and use on a daily basis.

Treating your entire family at the same time is crucial because parasites and especially pinworms are highly contagious. Wash all bedding and undergarments in the hottest water available on the last day of the six-day treatment. Wash your hands frequently, and teach your children to always wash their hands with soap after using the restroom, before eating, and whenever they are dirty. The practice of counting to 30 while washing their hands is a good way to insure that your children keep the water on long enough to get their hands clean. Keep your own and your children's fingernails trimmed short. If you have pets or animals, teach your children to avoid face-licking and to always wash their hands after playing with the dog or cat.

YEAST INFECTION

The mutation of candida into a fungal infection, or what is commonly known as yeast infection, is an unnecessary burden for the body to bear. After the parasite cleanse, if needed, add herbs to correct this condition during the second or third month of cleansing. **Pau D'Arco Bark, Licorice, Chamomile, Barberry** and **Oregon Grape Root** are used to control the proliferation of candida and to fight fungal infections. **Gotu Kola's** saponins have a weakening effect on membranous tissue making it easier for the above herbs to do their work. **Cat's Claw** cleanses and reduces inflammation in the entire gastrointestinal tract, while **Marshmallow** soothes irritation. **Ginger** neutralizes toxins, and **Sarsaparilla** binds off endotoxins who gain entry into the blood stream and facilitates their elimination from the body.

Since yeast infections are often difficult to eliminate. It is important to use the herbs for at least three months and for both partners to participate in the cleanse. Alternating two effective combinations every two weeks such as **Yeast X I** and **Yeast X II** can prevent developing immunity to the herbs. Die-off can cause headaches, nausea and increased itching during the initial stage of cleansing.

Sarsaparilla Root can keep the process more comfortable by binding to the endotoxins that gain entry into the blood stream and facilitating their elimination from the body. Don't be discouraged with this process! Instead, focus on drinking at least two quarts of water with fresh organic lemon daily, rest as needed, and be sure to replace the bad bacteria with beneficial bacteria found in probiotics. Avoid sugar, sugary drinks, and white flour. In their place, focus on fresh vegetables, nuts, and whole foods.

The length of time needed to thoroughly cleanse a yeast infection varies. Three months is a reasonable expectation for less severe cases. If the problem has been long- standing with frequent outbreaks over the years, or if the infection is present in the blood, the process will take longer. Be sure to rid yourself of parasites who can further complicate this condition. If you are a married couple, you both need to cleanse, even if only one of you has symptoms. By doing so, you will prevent the possibility of re-infection.

The benefits of cleansing are many, from a delightful feeling of refreshment to the disappearance of painful or uncontrollable symptoms. Among my favorite testimonies is a letter I received from an older Amish gentleman in Indiana who was able to lift a glass of water to his lips without spilling it after completing a whole body and colon cleanse. He was also delighted to be able to again hold his hymnbook and even share it with his neighbor without the shaking that used to keep him from participating.

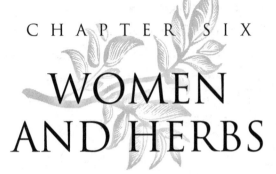

CHAPTER SIX

WOMEN AND HERBS

For centuries, women have used herbs to improve health and ease discomforts, and they have benefited in countless ways from these natural, God-given gifts. Today's modern woman is returning to an interest in knowing what herbs have to offer, and I am frequently asked, "But what can your herbs do for me as a woman?" To answer this important question, I first wanted to understand the leading causes of suffering and death among women. Once these were identifying, I journeyed into a study of available current research that demonstrates how herbal remedies can address and prevent unnecessary pain, suffering, and premature death in women.

CANCER

Breast cancer claims the lives of 196,000 women yearly in the United States alone. Most of these women are over 50 years of age. Since cancer cells can take as long as 15 years to develop, it makes sense to switch to a healthy lifestyle and use herbs as a preventative in your twenties or thirties, especially if you have a family history of this disease. **Propolis Resin** extract is high in Caffeic Acid Phenethyl Ester (CAPE) and may be helpful. Also, **Scullcap** has been studied and shown to increase the body's defense against cancer of various types including breast and skin. **Red Clover** enjoys a long history of application in fighting cancers and is now thought to inhibit the proliferation of breast and ovarian cancer cells.

Ovarian and cervical cancers take the lives of approximately another 32,000 women every year. Many of them are mothers who will leave behind grieving children and spouses. Here again, it makes sense to have and implement a prevention plan in the thirties as most cases are not being diagnosed before age 45. With excessive estrogen considered a contributor to most cancers of the female organs, it is very important to maintain a healthy hormone balance. For this, **Vitex Berry** shines as a normalizing herb that is not known to overcorrect any hormone. **False Unicorn, Blessed Thistle**, and **Squawvine** are all valuable female tonics. **Rosemary** counteracts the negative effects of certain estrogens. Inflammation is believed to contribute to cancer as well. **Olive Leaf, Astragulus, Ashwaganda,** and **Green Tea** reduce inflammation.

Liver and skin cancers also take a costly toll on women. **Milk Thistle Seed** extract is high in silymarin. It protects the liver by strengthening and stabilizing cell membranes. **Parsley Root** and **Nettle Leaf** are rich in minerals and vitamins. Together with chlorophyll, they rejuvenate red blood cells and accelerate the clearing of toxins from the liver. **Ashwaganda** and **Cat's Claw** are thought to inhibit skin cancer cells, protect the liver, and reduce inflammation. Because of its humulon content, **Hops Flower** extract is associated with the prevention of breast, colon, and skin cancer.

HEART DISEASE

Heart disease is another leading cause of death in women. **Hawthorn Berry** is very beneficial to the cardio-vascular system in alleviating angina and arrhythmias while improving the structural integrity of the arteries. **Gingko Biloba** deters abnormal blood clotting, making it useful in preventing stroke. This herb is also used to lower blood pressure and may prevent heart attacks. **Bilberry Fruit, Bilberry Leaf,** and **Ginger** work to improve blood circulation and lower blood pressure. **Olive Leaf** improves overall heart function.

FATIGUE

Fatigue has become a chief complaint among women, and Chronic Fatigue Syndrome has 500,000 women desperately searching for answers. **Sarsaparilla Root, Condonopsis**, and **Eleuthero** al-leviate fatigue and improve the body's ability to handle stress. **Licorice Root** and **Neem Leaf** contain powerful antioxidants to fight chronic fatigue. Licorice also stimulates adrenal hormone production. **Gingko Biloba Leaf** may alleviate fatigue as well as destroying free radicals and inactivating their formation. **Hops Flower** decreases the sensation of pain through its effect on the central nervous system.

OSTEOPOROSIS

Osteoporosis affects one of every four women over the age of 50. It reduces bone mass and causes the bones to become brittle and porous. The good news is that this aging problem is preventable. The bad news is that waiting until your late forties to implement a preventative plan is not wise. Regular **exercise** during the early adult years adds to bone mineral density and reduces bone loss during menopause. In clinical studies, **Progesterone cream** increased bone mass by up to 15 percent in postmenopausal women after three years of use by increasing osteoblast activity. **Calcium** and the minerals it needs to build and maintain strong bones, such as manganese, magnesium, and silicon, are readily available in plant matter and easily assimilated as liquid extracts. For a description of these herbs and **Herbal Calcium** please see Chapter Three.

FEMME DEFENSE FOR FEMALES

Our quest to discover which plants were most beneficial to women led to a combination of the 26 herbs discussed in the previous paragraphs with **Horsetail, Oat Straw, Cornsilk, Chamomile, and Mistletoe** included. The final product represents more than six months of careful, intense research and is named **Femme Defense**. Containing all the herbs found in **Herbal Calcium** and **Herbal CardioCare,** this all-in-one formulation is quick and easy to use on a daily basis and ideal for the busy mom who takes disease prevention seriously.

OVARIAN CYSTS

Ovarian cysts are often painless and symptomless, but they can contribute to infertility and, in some cases, can be extremely painful. For cysts as small as a marble or larger than a baseball, herbs are worth trying as an alternative to surgery. In just a matter of weeks, combinations such as the **T&C Formula,** which contains **False Unicorn** to normalize follicular development and female organ tonics such as **Red Raspberry, Mistletoe, Blue Cohosh,** and **Blessed Thistle** have helped women avoid an operation. When choosing an appropriate herbal combination, be sure it includes **Yarrow** to clear congestion. **Progesterone cream** is also valuable here, as estrogen dominance is thought to be the underlying cause of cysts including polycystic ovary syndrome. **Calcium** is also essential to ovarian health and will go a long way in relieving the pain.

Painful ovulation, or the discomfort experienced at mid-cycle due to ovulation, can be eased with the correct herbs. Since **calcium** is essential to the health of the ovaries, effective treatment may be as simple as adding this supplement to the diet and increasing the intake from day 12 through day 16 or whenever the discomfort arises. **False Unicorn's** bitter compounds reduce ovarian swelling and inflammation. They also enhance the overall function of the ovaries and can be taken throughout the cycle or as needed. Avoid MSG, which can cause atrophy or a decrease in the size of the ovaries.

MORE HB FORMULA BENEFITS

Hormone-related acne and irregular cycles can be a huge source of frustration for teenage girls, but relief can be found in the correct combination of herbs that support hormonal balance and blood purification. **Chaste Tree Berry** has a normalizing effect on estrogen and FSH levels while stimulating the production of progesterone. **Sarsaparilla Root** cleanses the blood and is included in formulations designed to balance hormones and address inflammatory skin conditions. **Blessed Thistle** and **Squawvine** are used by herbalists to relieve painful menstruation. They also contain astringent, antiseptic compounds that shrink inflamed issue. **Ginger Root** purifies the blood, which in turn, clears the skin. **False Unicorn Root** reduces swelling and inflammation; its bitter compounds enhance ovarian function and bring balance to female hormone levels.

MENOPAUSE

Menopause challenges older women with a variety of symptoms including night sweats, heavy bleeding, hot flashes and insomnia. However, the right herbs can make this life transition much smoother and certainly less miserable. **Progesterone cream** can help correct the hormonal imbalance creating many of these symptoms. **Sage** and **Calcium** can relieve night sweats when additional support is needed. Heavy bleeding can be controlled with a combination of **Crampbark, Lady's Mantle, Yarrow, Bayberry, Barberry,** and **Shepherd's Purse**.

In one study, taking 1,200 mg daily of **Vitamin C** for eight weeks along with **St. John's Wort** reduced hot flashes in menopausal women. **Chaste Tree Berry** and **False Unicorn** can help normalize hormone levels, the underlying cause of most hot flashes. **Tribulus Terrestris** may alleviate the typical anxiety, insomnia, irritability, and depression associated with menopause. Decreased libido or lack of sexual desire is common in menopausal women, **Progesterone Cream**, **Tribulus Terrestris, Gingko Biloba,** and **Gotu Kola** can increase the hormones associated with libido.

INSOMNIA

Although menopausal insomnia is common, you can still learn how to enjoy a good night of deep restful sleep naturally. Brewing a pot of after-dinner tea containing relaxing herbs such as catnip, chamomile, lemon balm, and spearmint is a great way to start unwinding. **Valerian Root** acts as a soother and depressant of the central nervous system. High in calcium, it has a very calming effect. **Hops** acts as a mild sedative and is often combined with Valerian. **Passionflower** can relieve restlessness, irritability, and difficulty falling asleep. **Scullcap** also contains sedative properties and is used to treat insomnia. Taking a liquid extract combination of these herbs twenty minutes before bedtime and repeating the dosage as needed, can make the difference between a miserable night and a restful one for the menopausal women.

Interestingly, an added benefit of taking **Herbal Calcium** throughout the day is more restful, restorative sleep at night.

CHAPTER SEVEN

HERBS AND CHILDREN

L iquid Herbal extracts are fast-acting and very easy for children to ingest. The educated, well-prepared mom can ward off illness and ease symptoms in many cases, without leaving her home to make an exhausting trip to the doctor. While it is important to remember that what is appropriate for an adult can harm a child, especially one who is under the age of two, nature does have many wonderful, effective herbs for little ones that are perfectly safe to use. Do your homework before illness strikes, and have a supply ready to battle the issues your children face most often. An excellent in-depth resource on herbs and children is *Mommy Diagnostics* by herbalist Shonda Parker.

Elderberry extract is the first thing I reach for when my little ones seem to be coming down with something. With the H1N1 swine flu scare adding to the usual concern each cold season brings, last winter, I took the extra step of giving them elderberry glycerite on a daily basis to keep them healthy. Research showing its antiviral activity against multiple strains of influenza increased my confidence, and in spite of travel and exposure, we made it through the winter with no trips to the doctor and only one mild case of fever, sore throat, and coughing. **Elderberry** can be safely given to infants and is great for adults as well.

Only the most benign herbs are appropriate for infants. With this having been said, **Chamomile** and **Catnip** have been used by moms for centuries to calm and soothe their babies. In a 1993 study, a tea containing **Chamomile** alleviated colic in 57 percent of infants. **Catnip** is relaxing and stimulates digestion. **Fennel** seed is also used to relieve colic and gas in infants. Rather than making a tea while the crying continues and hoping to get your little one to drink it, simply place a few drops of a combination of these extracts, made with glycerine and distilled water, into your baby's mouth. Although an allergic response is rare, always observe your infant carefully for any reaction or change in breathing, and do not exceed the suggested dosage. **Infant Tummy Aid**

Unresolved diarrhea is dangerous, especially in young children and infants. If the diarrhea is flu-related and your child is running a fever and vomiting, it is especially important to stop the diarrhea as soon as possible to avoid dehydration. **Ginger** root has a direct and immediate effect on the stomach and digestive system, and the tannins in **Red Raspberry** leaf firms up loose stools while providing pectin, folic acid, and vitamin A. **Bayberry's** tannins are astringent in nature, and the berberine in **Barberry** fights several types of detrimental bacteria, which can be the underlying cause of the problem. This combination of herbs, **Anti-Diarrhea,** has repeatedly stopped diarrhea with only one dose. I don't travel anywhere without it. **Barberry** should not be given to children under two. **Propolis Resin, Olive Leaf** and **Elderberry** are safer options.

Teething misery in babies can be eased with **Herbal Calcium**. In addition to calming the fussy little one, it helps meet the demands placed on the body by tooth formation. Teeth are mainly made up of calcium, magnesium and silicon. **Horsetail,** the most bio-available form of silicon used by the body to produce collagen another important part of strong healthy teeth. For a more complete description of **Herbal Calcium**, what is in it and its benefits, see page 28.

A strong, healthy immune system is built, in part, during childhood as germs, viruses, and bacteria are fought off and immunity is built. Antibiotics may fight invaders, but they do nothing to help strengthen your child's own resistance to disease. In fact, much damage is done to friendly microorganisms, and your child is left with less rather than more resistance. Herbs such as **Echinacea,** to the contrary, will strengthen the body's natural defenses while attacking invaders. When both **Echinacea Purpurea** and the root of **Echinacia Augustofolia** are combined with **Elderberry** and **Propolis** resin extract, a powerful, infant-safe herbal remedy is created to fight flus and colds. Using **Infant Immune Booster,** which contains the extracts of these herbs, or a similar combination, will increase your child's resistance rather than lessening it.

Infant earaches can keep mom and her baby up all night, an experience that should definitely add at least one more star to any mother's crown. This experience understandably , will often take most moms straight to the doctor's office, where the cycle of antibiotics begins. For some, surgery to place tubes in the ears is the next step. It doesn't have to end this way. **Propolis Resin** extract, **Elderberry,** and both **Echinaceas** are well worth trying on an ongoing basis before submitting your child to surgery or antibiotics. Avoid getting water in the ears. Instead of washing hair in the tub, lay your child on the countertop and use the sink. For a few minutes, heat a bit of **olive oil** as you rub peeled garlic clove in it. Insert a drop or two of the warm oil in the ear to provide immediate relief from the pain and to help fight the infection. A bit of cotton placed in the ear to protect it after the drops are inserted will keep the child comfortable longer. Make sure everything used, including your hands and the dropper, are very clean.

A FEVER IS YOUR BODY'S FRIEND

Fever is part of the body's natural mechanism to fight invading organisms. Since it is a symptom of underlying illness, a fever is the signal to bring out the herbs that work best to stimulate and support the immune system and to fight the illness. Fevers of less than 102 degrees are usually not dangerous, and most children are fairly comfortable until their temperature exceeds this number. I tend to allow a fever to do its work unless my child is very uncomfortable or the temperature reading exceeds 102.5 degrees, at which time vomiting seems to start. For infants, **Elderflower** extract has been found to be helpful in reducing fever. **Ginger** can be added for older children and adults. American Indians used **Bayberry** for the same purpose. Increase liquid intake (water is best) and dress the child in cool, loose-fitting clothing until the episode subsides.

Children's tonsils used to be routinely removed if inflammation, swelling, and infections were frequent; however, today, these little glands are recognized as an important part of the immune system. Sitting at the back of the throat, they trap and block bacteria and other invaders from penetrating deeper into the body. "B" and "T" lymphocytes are stored in the tonsils until they are needed by the immune system. A liquid combination of herbs will affect the tonsils topically as the remedy is being swallowed before entering the blood stream.

Our daughter suffered from frequent bouts of severe tonsillitis. Pockets of pus were clearly visible, and in spite of using the immune boosting herbs that worked so well for her brothers, she ended up on antibiotics. I knew I could do better for her. So, after more research, I created a combination of the following herbs and gave them to her at the first hint of sore throat. **White Oak** bark and **Slippery Elm** both contain tannins used to relieve tonsillitis, sore throat, and loss of voice. **Propolis, Olive Leaf,** and **Oregon Grape Root** combat many of the bacteria and viruses that cause sore throat and tonsillitis. **Devil's Claw** can be used to reduce inflammation and swelling and ease the pain of swallowing. It worked very well for her and others. We named it **Heidi's Tonsil Formula** and it is still available from Mountain Meadow Herbs. This combination should not be used for extended periods of time and is not appropriate for infants.

Ridding your little one of parasites can make the difference between a pale, tired, irritable child who only wants to eat bread and sweets and a healthy, happy child who enjoys healthy, whole foods. Teeth grinding at night, abdominal pain, frequent illness, and itching of the anus are other signs that your child can benefit from a good herbal parasite cleanse. For children under the age of two, **Olive Leaf** extract is the best choice. For older children, a combination containing **Wormwood, Black Walnut Hulls** and **Cloves** along with herbs to make the cleansing process more comfortable, such as those in **Para-Rid,** is an excellent choice. Parasites are discussed in more detail in Chapter Five.

Respiratory infections in children can often be resolved with herbal remedies, especially if treatment begins as soon as the coughing or fever is noticed. **Thyme Leaf** is a powerful bronchial antispasmodic and expectorant used to loosen chest congestion and relieve coughing. **Elecampane** is an expectorant and contains compounds that are antibiotic and antimicrobial. **Anise Seed** extract is used to loosen mucous and relieve coughing. **Nettle Leaf** and **Elderflower** inhibit the replication of some influenza viruses, **Nettle** can also relieve coughing caused by allergies. **Licorice Root** acts as an anti-inflammatory, expectorant, and antibacterial agent. **Bayberry Bark** is used to relieve symptoms of the common cold. A combination of these herbs, **Herbal Respiratory,** can significantly help maintain open, unrestricted airways without introducing the side effects of drug-laced cough syrups and decongestants.

If your child suffers from asthma begin with a thorough parasite cleanse. The connection between asthma and roundworms is too well-documented to ignore. To ensure healing and strengthening, support your child's respiratory system for a few weeks following the cleanse with a combination of herbs such as those in **Herbal Respiratory.** Interestingly, eczema and skin rashes in children can be parasitical in nature, and children who suffer from eczema often go on to develop asthma. Researcher Dr. Clark has found both of these conditions and other skin problems to be caused by the same parasite, the roundworm.

Attention Deficit Disorder (ADD) causes children to find focusing and concentrating on a task for more than a few minutes impossible. These children easily become anxious, forgetful, fidgety, impatient, and hyperactive. Regardless of the setting, it is hard for them to be at peace. It is estimated that as many as 20 percent of the school-age children in the USA are afflicted with ADD. The condition is more prevalent among males than females by a ratio of approximately 4-to-1. In this country, drugs are widely used to control the symptoms and to help children fit into their environments more appropriately.

There are four simple herbs that can transform the behavior of a child faced with this challenge. **American Ginseng** root extract relieves anxiety, calms nervousness, and improves learning. **Gingko Biloba** boosts blood and oxygen circulation to the brain, increasing concentration and mental function. **Valerian** root is very calming. It is used to eliminate the restlessness, fear, and aggression associated with ADD and to improve coordination. Attention span can be increased and learning and memory improved with **Gotu Kola. Natural Attention Aid.**

Four simple herbs can transform the behavior of a child faced with the challenge of ADD.

Calcium deficiency is also thought to contribute to ADD, it is very important that your child take an easily absorbed calcium supplement on a daily basis.

Growing pains are a sign that your child is growing rapidly. They are also a sure indicator of calcium deficiency. These pains can be easily and almost immediately relieved with **Herbal Calcium**, but to help your child develop strong bones don't wait for the growing pains to alert you to the deficiency. Daily supplementation is especially important for little girls. Recent research shows the risk for osteoporosis later in life is connected to the degree of bone calcification before the onset of menstruation. Be sure the supplement you chose is easily assimilated and from natural food sources or herbs rather than from oyster shells or coral calcium. In addition to being difficult for the body to use, these are often contaminated with unwanted heavy metals.

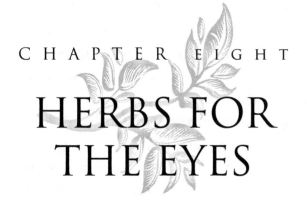

CHAPTER EIGHT

HERBS FOR THE EYES

Seeing is such a big part of everyday life. In fact, nearly half of the brain gets involved in the process. Our eyes may look like simple orbs, but in reality, they are amazing and highly complex organs. Eye cells are very unique in purpose and shape. For example, cone-shaped cells allow you to see color while rod-shaped cells help you distinguish shapes and shades of color. With more than two million working parts, eye muscles are the body's most active muscle group.

There are seven main parts to the eye. Each one plays an important role in sending information to the brain, detecting light, and focusing. A problem in any of these parts causes a vision issue. While we are young, little thought is given to how valuable it is to be able to see well, but as we mature, the years begin to take their toll on our bodies. For most of us, as our eyesight declines, we suddenly realize that seeing has been a very precious gift—one well worth protecting.

As we age, it is common for reading glasses to become a necessity. Small print becomes difficult to read, and the newspaper must be held at arm's length to be enjoyed. Age-related macular degeneration in those 65 years of age or older is responsible for much of the blurring and loss of sharp central vision that is so necessary for reading, pursuing hobbies, and driving. Unfortunately, the problem can begin as early as the mid-to-late forties and can gradually worsen as the years pass. By the late seventies, a familiar face may be unrecognizable unless it is seen up close. The National Eye Institute cites this painless degeneration of the macula, one of the seven main parts of the eye, as the leading cause of vision loss in Americans over age 60. This painless process destroys the macula, the part of the eye that helps you see fine detail.

While the exact causes of failing eyesight are not all clearly understood, damage to the blood vessels of the eye, the presence of abnormal blood vessels, and poor blood supply to the eyes are thought to be big contributors to the problem. High blood pressure, diabetes, and obesity are considered risk factors, as is having a family member who has experienced serious vision loss. It is important to know your family eye history and to maintain a healthy weight, especially if there is a history of diabetes in your family.

Another way to protect your vision is to avoid rubbing your eyes excessively. This habit can damage the cornea, the clear front covering, or window of the eye that allows light to enter and begins the refractory process of sending images to the retina. The rest of your body can tolerate a lot of scarring with little damage done, but not the cornea. Even a minor scar or irregularity in its shape can impair vision. No matter how well the rest of the eye is functioning, if the cornea is scarred, clouded, or distorted, your vision will be affected. If you have ongoing allergies or eye floaters, consider doing a good intestinal and parasite cleanse.

A COMMON CHEMICAL THAT DAMAGES EYESIGHT

Sodium laureth sulfite travels to and concentrates in the cornea of the eye. Once there, it damages eye proteins and prevents healing and cell regeneration. This chemical is commonly found in shampoos and body washes, even those designated for babies. It is included as a foaming or bubbling agent because we have all grown accustomed to the idea that a soap or shampoo needs to produce lather to clean well. Sodium laureth sulfite does not have to come in contact with your eyes for damage to occur; it readily permeates the skin or scalp and then travels to the eyes.

Choose bar soap containing natural ingredients instead of body washes, and read your shampoo label. There are shampoos available without sodium laureth sulfite, although most of them in my experience do not suds up as well as the brands containing it. Dr. Bonner's castile soaps are a great choice, as are the Sanctum personal care products. Just keep in mind that bubbles and lather are not imperative to being clean.

Keep your liver in great health too because much of what your body uses for eye repair is stored in the liver. Fat-soluble vitamins are stored and released by the liver and B vitamins are activated here. Interestingly enough, the liver is another organ that sodium laureth sulfite travels to and concentrates in. Choose a diet rich in plant matter, and yes, spinach is good for you! A NIH Eye Disease Case–Control study done in 1995 found that eating spinach or collard greens five times a week significantly reduced the risk of vision loss.

Opinions on the best herbs for the eyes vary; however, most begin with or include **Bilberry** and **Eyebright** in the herbal products used to reduce inflammation and to increase blood flow to the eyes. Bilberry jam was reportedly eaten by British pilots to improve night vision during World War II. **Bilberry** is the most studied herb related to eye health. It has been tested in the treatment of many eye ailments including glaucoma, retinopathy, poor night vision, work-related eye fatigue, age-related macular degeneration, and eye inflammation. **Bilberry's** anthocyanosides are thought to alleviate many eye conditions simply by increasing blood flow to the eyes, strengthening and stabilizing eye capillaries, and improving blood circulation in the retina. **Eyebright** flowers resemble the eyes, and this herb enjoys a long history of traditional use as a natural vision support.

Ginkgo Biloba is used to increase blood circulation to the optic nerve in particular and is an increasingly popular part of most herbal combinations used to support crisp, clear central vision. Inflammation can compress the optic nerve, causing serious vision loss and distortion, but **Gentian, Tumeric,** and **Ginger Root** extracts are great natural anti- inflammatory agents for optimal eye health. The OPCs found in **Grape Seed** extract reduce free radical damage in the eyes. A 1978 study involving the use of 100 mgs of OPCs from grape seeds showed improvement in 147 diabetic retinopathy patients. **Grape Seed** extract is also used to reduce bright light sensitivity.

Propolis Resin extract, a honey bee product, has a significant neuroprotective effect on the retina. As a powerful antioxidant, it helps to mend and protect the retina from oxidative damage. Michael T. Murray in *The Power of Healing Herbs* notes that the OPC content of **Hawthorn Berry** preserves the integrity of collagen structures within the body. Collagen is an important structural component of the eyes. The sclera (the tissue that makes up the white of the eye) is all collagen and represents 80 percent of the eye. The cornea is mostly collagen as well.

Eleuthero can support light and color perception, while **Schizandra** extract can help extend the eye's visual field. In spite of its long history of being a great herb for the eyes, **Eyebright** has not been studied extensively, and little in the form of scientific study proves it to be beneficial to the eyes. However, Aucubin, a constituent of Eyebright has been shown to positively affect the liver. Some claim its cleansing action on the liver releases stored Vitamin A, which in turn, benefits the eyes. Given its long history and high status among modern herbalists, it seems wise to include this respected herb in a well-rounded herbal vision support. **Eye-Can-C**

Coenzyme Q 10 is found in every cell of the human body, including the eyes. However, patients with age-related macular degeneration have lower levels of this important fat- soluble quinone. Studies indicate CoQ10 is useful in the treatment and prevention of glaucoma by counteracting the toxicity of glutamic acid, a suspected cause of glaucoma. The authors of a 2010 study concluded that Coenzyme Q10 may help prevent cataracts by significantly reducing light-induced LEC damage that leads to cataracts. The suggested dosage is 180 – 300 mgs per day.

Vitamins A, C, E, and **B2** also contribute to the structural integrity and health of the eyes. Taking a reputable brand multivitamin made from natural food sources is a good idea to help maintain and protect your vision. Choose a product that contains 2 mgs of copper and 80 mgs of zinc, as these micronutrients are especially important when dealing with age- related macular degeneration.

What you eat can have a very positive impact on your eye health. Take a few minutes to look over these delicious foods, they are a literal feast for your eyes. Then make plans to include more of them in your diet. It is well worth the effort to protect one of life's most precious gifts.

"EYE-FRIENDLY" FOODS

tomatoes	pomegranates	whole grains
apples	peaches	cauliflower
watermelon	Brussel sprouts	lemons
pineapple	olives	spinach
mustard greens	nectarines	cabbage
garlic	tuna	asparagus
avocado	grapefruit	carrots

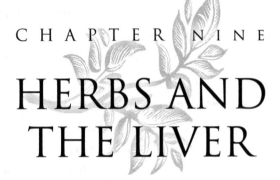

CHAPTER NINE

HERBS AND
THE LIVER

The word "liver" means life. It is not called the *"live-r"* for nothing—it keeps us living! Second in size only to the skin, it is approximately 2.5 percent of body weight. This is an important organ, and its maintenance is considered to be foundational to vibrant health. Processing an impressive three pints of blood per minute around the clock, it sits under the rib cage slightly on the right side of the body. As the primary organ of detoxification, the liver also participates in the function of the cardiovascular, digestive/metabolic, and excretory systems.

Responsible for 25 percent of basal metabolism, the liver takes raw materials from food such as proteins, carbohydrates, and fats and breaks them down into basic components used to create and store glycogen. Glycogens are used as both immediate and long-term energy sources. A congested liver restricts the flow/production of bile and can cause jaundice, indigestion, and bloating.

Detoxification of toxic chemicals that enter the body is done by the liver. When overloaded by stress or prescription drugs, it stores toxins rather than processing and eliminating them. Additionally, new chemicals are approved and added to our food supply each year, further stressing this important organ. If the liver is sluggish, excessive amounts of toxic metabolites find their way into the blood stream. Bilirubin, the yellow pigment produced when red blood cells die (via bile), is also cleansed from the blood by the liver. Blood is stored in the liver and infectious organisms are filtered out. When the liver is diseased or congested, not enough blood is sent or received, and your energy, along with your mood, drops.

According to traditional Chinese medicine, which also considers negative emotions a hindrance to optimal liver function, a healthy liver helps maintain an even temperament. Symptoms of a liver needing help can include:

- Feeling blue
- Foggy brain
- Depression
- Fatigue
- Indigestion
- Bloating

- Unpleasant mood changes
- Poor concentration and memory
- Pain in the liver area
- Shoulder pain and upper arm pain
- Gallstones
- Jaundice

Liver-friendly herbs are readily available. **Ginger, Alfalfa, Dandelion,** and **Yellow Dock** have a cleansing effect. **Gentian, Quassia, Oregon Grape** root, and **Lemon Balm** are used to stimulate the liver and increase bile production. **Alfalfa, Oatstraw,** and **Blessed Thistle** are nourishing and build up the liver. **Milk Thistle, Grape Seed extract, Olive Leaf**, and **Bilberry** are used to protect the liver. These herbs are particularly effective in liquid extract form in a combination such as **LiverGlow** when used for three months to enhance liver health.

During the first month of use, do a parasite cleanse because it is difficult to cleanse the liver if parasites are present, and some invaders do take up residence in the liver. After completing the parasite cleanse, use a **liver flush** to decongest and unclog the liver bile ducts. This liver and gallbladder flush comes to us from Dr. Hulda Clark who considers it to be the most powerful procedure one can do to improve health.

LIVER AND GALLBLADDER FLUSH

- Mix 4 tablespoons Epsom salts with 1/2 (one-half) cup olive oil (Light olive oil is easier to get down).

- Add 2/3 (two-thirds) cup juice squeezed from 1 large or 2 small fresh pink grapefruits. Wash whole fruit in hot water twice first, and dry each time.

- Take 4–8 Ornithine capsules to help you sleep. Don't skip this, or you may have the worst night of your life!

- Use a large plastic straw to help drink potion.

- Take 10–20 drops of Black Walnut Tincture, any strength, to kill parasites coming from the liver.

- Choose a day like Saturday for the cleanse so you will be able to rest the next day.

During this time, take no medicines, vitamins, or pills that you can do without. They could prevent success. Stop the parasite program and kidney herbs too on the day before you start. Eat a no-fat breakfast and lunch. You may have cooked cereal, fruit, fruit juice, bread, and preserves or honey (no butter or milk). This allows the bile to build up and develop pressure in the liver. Higher pressure pushes out more stones.

On the day of your cleanse ...

- **2:00 p.m.** Do not eat or drink after 2 p.m. If you break this rule, you could feel quite ill later. Get your Epsom salts ready. Mix 4 tbs. in 3 cups water and pour this into a jar.

  This makes four servings, 3/4 (three-fourths) cup each. Set the jar in the refrigerator to get ice cold (this is for convenience and taste only).

- **6:00 p.m.** Drink one 3/4 (three-fourths cup) serving of the ice-cold Epsom salts. If you did not prepare this ahead of time, mix 1 tbs. in 3/4 (three-fourths) cup water now. You may add 1/8 (one- eighth) tsp. vitamin C powder to improve the taste. You may also drink a few mouthfuls of water afterwards or rinse your mouth. Get the olive oil and grapefruit out to warm up.

- **8:00 p.m.** Repeat by drinking another 3/4 (three-fourths) cup of Epsom salts. You haven't eaten since two o'clock, but you won't feel hungry. Get your bedtime chores done. The proper timing is critical for success.

- **9:45 p.m.** Pour 1/2 (one-half) cup (measured) olive oil into the pint jar. Add 2 drops HCl to sterilize. Wash grapefruit twice in hot water and dry; squeeze juice by hand into the measuring cup. Remove pulp with fork. You should have at least 1/2 (one-half) cup, or more. Up to 3/4 (three-fourths) cup is best. You may use part lemonade. Add the juice to the olive oil. Also add Black Walnut Tincture. Close the jar tightly with the lid, and shake hard until watery. Only fresh grapefruit juice produces this effect. Now visit the bathroom one or more times, even if it makes you late for your ten o'clock drink, but don't be more than 15 minutes late. Your liver will release fewer stones if you wait too long.

- **10:00 p.m.** Drink the potion you have mixed. Take 4 Ornithine capsules with the first sips to make sure you will sleep through the night. Take 8 if you already suffer from insomnia. Drinking through a large plastic straw helps this concoction go down easier. You may also use oil and vinegar salad dressing, or straight honey to chase it down between sips. Have these ready in a tablespoon on the kitchen counter. Take everything to your bedside if you want, but drink standing up. Get the drink down within 5 minutes (fifteen minutes for very elderly or weak persons).

Lie down immediately (you might fail to get stones out if you don't). The sooner you lie down, the more stones that can be released. Prepare for bed ahead of time. Don't clean up the kitchen. As soon as the drink is down, walk to your bed and lie down flat on your back with your head up high on a pillow. Try to think about what is happening in the liver, and try to keep perfectly still for at least 20 minutes. You may feel a train of stones traveling along the bile ducts like rolling marbles. There is no pain because the bile duct valves are open (thank you, Epsom salts!). Go to sleep. Once again, you may fail to get stones out if you don't.

- **Next morning.** Upon waking, take your third dose of Epsom salts. If you have indigestion or nausea, wait until that passes before drinking the Epsom salts. You may go back to bed. **Do not** take this potion before 6:00 a.m.

- **2 hours later.** Take your fourth (the last) dose of Epsom salts. You may go back to bed again.

- **After 2 more hours,** you may eat. Start with fruit juice. Half an hour later eat fruit. One hour later you may eat regular food, but keep the content light. Expect diarrhea in the morning. By dinner you should feel recovered. Dr. Clark recommends this flush as very safe; however, it should never be done during illness.

Liver flushes vary in intensity. You have options to try this healthy process.

Liver flushes vary in intensity, with Dr. Clark's being among the most intense. A gentler option is to mix **1 cup of freshly squeezed grapefruit and lemon juice.** Add **1-2 freshly squeezed cloves** of **Garlic** and **one teaspoon of fresh Ginger Root juice.** This can easily be made by grating the ginger and pressing the fiber in a garlic press.

Add **1 tablespoon of extra virgin olive oil**. Blend or shake well and drink every morning before breakfast for ten days. Follow with a cup or two of liver-cleansing tea, and wait one hour to eat breakfast. This flush can be repeated after a rest of three to five days.

LIVER-CLEANSING TEA FORMULAS

Liver-cleansing teas should contain herbs that have a strong opening and decongesting effect on the bile ducts while increasing bile production. **Polari Tea** and the **Liver Decongestant Tea** recommended by Dr. Christopher Hobbs are good options, as is the **Puri-Tea** by herbalist Brigitte Mars. These teas can be found in some health foods stores. Mountain Meadow Herbs carries a Liver Decongestant Tea sold as **Liver Cleansing Tea.** It contains **Burdock Root, Dandelion Root, Fennel, Ginger Root, Mugwort Herb, and Milk Thistle Seed**.

Garlic is also very liver friendly. Use it liberally in cooking, and if your digestion is poor, add garlic tablets. Garlic contains important sulfuric compounds used by the liver to build enzymes. It may facilitate the ability of the liver to detoxify chemicals before they can exert their harmful effects within the body. Choose fresh, organic, liver-friendly fruits and vegetables from spring and summer's bounty. Cabbage is among the most beneficial choices. Freshly ground flax seeds make a great addition to muffins, pancakes, and hot cereals. A small coffee grinder is perfect for grinding. Flax seed and flax-seed oil are used to improve liver function and to protect this valuable organ.

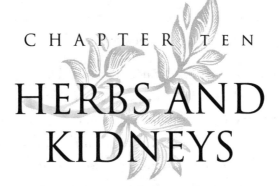

C H A P T E R   T E N

HERBS AND KIDNEYS

The kidneys are bean-shaped organs, each about the size of a fist. Located near the middle of the back and just below the rib cage, one sits on each side of the spine. As sophisticated re-processing machines, your kidneys process 200 quarts of blood by sifting out about two quarts of waste products and extra water every day. Blood filtration is done by the nephrons within the cortex and medulla or the kidney wall. Waste and extra water (urine) collect in the center of the kidney and then flow to the bladder through the ureters. When the nephrons are compromised by disease, injury, or toxic substances, their job cannot be properly done. Kidney function decreases, and wastes build up, damaging the body.

Common causes of kidney damage include diabetes, high blood pressure, polycystic kidney disease, and genetic and autoimmune disorders, all of which attack the nephrons. Since we are born with about one million nephrons per kidney, life can be lived quite normally with only 30 to 40 percent kidney function. However, when healthy function drops below 15 percent, intervention becomes necessary. Usually dialysis and transplant are the only options presented.

In our son Tristan's case, an undetected blockage caused the collection area of the kidneys to expand as the pressure from the blocked urine increased and the wall containing the nephrons was compressed, becoming thinner and thinner under the pressure. Frequent urinary-tract infections added to the damage, and a severe kidney infection and dehydration landed him in the hospital again in 1997. At that time, he had very little remaining kidney function.

Tristan was still very weak and ill as we carried him out of the hospital, but in fact, a partial miracle had happened. Overnight, there had been enough improvement to avoid the surgery scheduled for the next morning. Over the next 10 days, his kidney function improved from two percent to 15 percent, which was just above dialysis level! While the specialist assured us that given the state of his kidneys, the improvement would not last more than a few months, I was determined to find a way to avoid dialysis.

I had no idea where to start in finding a way to help Tristan, but Nathan and I could not bring ourselves to accept dialysis as his only hope for survival. I turned to my faith and asked God to teach me and to make Tristan hungry for foods that would help him most in recovering. My confidence was boosted by the fact that just three months earlier I had heard my heavenly Father say

We could not bring ourselves to accept dialysis as Tristan's only hope for survival.

I would be the mother of children. Despite being told by a fertility specialist there would be no more babies, we were now expecting our second child!

With this encouragement, I started working on a solution for my son. My first impression was to give Tristan **garlic.** I ground tablets, mixed them in applesauce, and persuaded him to eat this three times a day. For several months, Tristan asked for **blueberries and oatmeal** two to three times a day. Fortunately, we had picked the berries together that summer on a beautiful mountainside overlooking the river, and we had filled the freezer. Months later, as I poured over herbal and nutritional volumes, science confirmed that my prayers had been heard and answered. Blueberries and oatmeal are both nourishing to the kidneys and can lower blood pressure.

HERBAL CARDIOCARE FOR HIGH BLOOD PRESSURE

Garlic has been clinically proven to lower blood pressure in as little as seven days by improving blood circulation, blood vessel strength, and elasticity. It is also used to promote urine production and excretion and may also stimulate the appetite, which was desperately needed in Tristan's case. The blueberry family is a wonderful natural gift when it comes to lowering blood pressure. However, I found **Bilberry** fruit and leaf extract to be more effective than eating blueberries. **Hawthorn Berry** lowers blood pressure by dilating the blood vessels and functioning as a diuretic. I added **Ginger** root, **Ginkgo Biloba,** and **Gotu Kola** extract for their ability to lower blood pressure and improve heart function.

This combination of herbs, known as **Herbal CardioCare,** is still available from Mountain Meadow Herbs in the exact formulation I created for Tristan.

As I continued searching, I discovered **Coenzyme Q10.** Found in every cell of the body, this nutrient is widely used as a supplement to support heart health and to lower blood pressure by normalizing the body's sodium/potassium ratio. I immediately added Coenzyme Q10 to Tristan's regime and added **Grape Seed** extract to minimize any free radical damage. **Capsicum** capsules were also added as soon as he could swallow pills. Within two weeks of taking what would become our **Herbal CardioCare, Coenzyme Q10, Grape Seed** extract, and **Garlic,** we walked hand in hand out of the doctor's office smiling—no more adult blood pressure medication for this little boy!

In searching for answers to improve Tristan's kidney function, I was overwhelmed more than once by the beauty of the Creator's wisdom and provision. Repeatedly, I found the same herbs or supplements such as Coenzyme Q10 to have a positive effect not only on blood pressure but also on kidney function. A randomized, double-blind, placebo-controlled study found that administering 60 mg of Coenzyme Q10 three times daily reduced the frequency of kidney dialysis after four weeks of treatment. Creatine and blood urea nitrogen levels (used to measure renal function) were significantly reduced, and there was a marked increase in creatine clearance and urine output. Like Coenzyme Q10, **Gingko Biloba** is another example of an herb that is beneficial to both kidney and cardiovascular health.

When using herbs to improve chronic conditions, it is best to alternate between two combinations and to give frequent small doses rather than one or two large ones. To prevent Tristan's kidneys from building immunity to specific herbs, I chose two combinations of liquid extracts to alternate on a bimonthly basis. The first combination was a bit stronger and more of a stimulating, cleansing formula, while the second one was more of a supportive tonic. It made sense to not over-stimulate his damaged kidneys, just as it is prudent not to whip a tired horse into running even faster. I avoided the stronger kidney stimulants such as Juniper Berry, Uva Ursi, and Gravel Root.

Parsley Root stimulates urine production/flow and relieves various urinary tract ailments. **Cornsilk** has not been well-studied, but is widely used to alleviate edema, painful urination, and kidney ailments. **Marshmallow Root** is soothing to irritated, inflamed mucous membranes. **Cleavers** is diuretic and stringent in nature. **Shepherd's Purse** is used in China to clear blood in urine and to stimulate urine flow. **Buchu Leaf**'s diuretic effect is used to flush bacteria from the urinary tract and may be helpful in flushing kidney stones. For relieving edema, **Blue Vervain** is astringent and anti-inflammatory. This combination of herbs has a stimulating and cleansing effect on the kidneys. **Kidney Toning Formula**

Dandelion Root is used to regulate the kidneys and as a normalizing tonic. **Milk Thistle** may stimulate the regeneration of kidney cells. **Sarsaparilla** is used to enhance kidney health and stimulate urine production. I added **Eleuthero** to this second combination because I hoped its adaptogenic effects would decrease the stress on his damaged kidneys. This herb is also thought to increase the production of red blood cells. **Kidney Support**

Healthy kidneys produce erythropoietin, a hormone that stimulates the production of red blood cells within bone marrow. When kidney function decreases, this hormone is no longer released, and anemia becomes a serious issue. Modern medicine treats the problem with a genetically engineered form of erythropoietin that is frequently poorly tolerated by the patient. Since my patient was my son, I chose the extracts of **Dandelion Root, Yellow Dock Root,** and **Stinging Nettle Leaf** instead. **Herbal Iron**

Raw garlic is also helpful in treating anemia. It can be pressed and then blended with pure orange-juice concentrate to mask the taste. If the issue of anemia becomes severe, Iron Plus Herbs from Floradix can be added.

Tristan's blockage caused severe structural damage to his entire urinary system, and its anomalies became the breeding ground for frequent, severe urinary-tract infections. Prevention was, and still is, a major focus. Anyone who has experienced a kidney infection will understand how heartbreaking it was for me to watch my child suffer through the pain and shaking. Since infection further damages nephrons, it is very important to stop it as soon as possible, especially if the kidneys are already compromised. I have not been able to find a non-antibiotic means beyond prayer to overcome these infections.

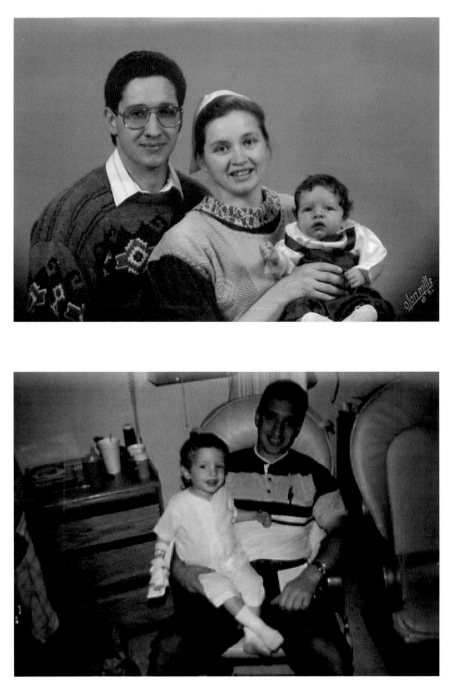

Tristan used to hide his arm with the I.V. in under his blanket as a nurse or doctor walked into the room. We spent Christmas Day, 1996 in The Children's Hospital in Kansas City

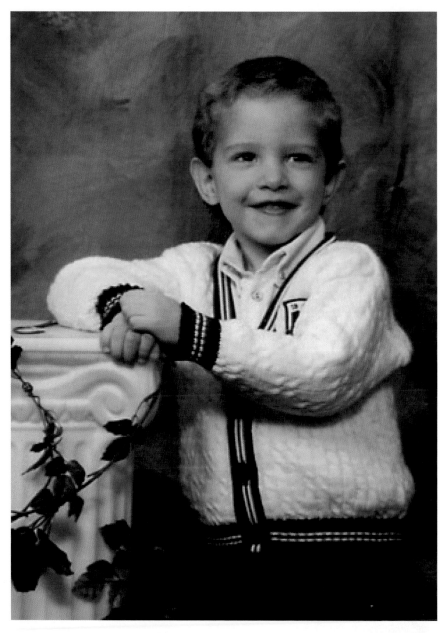

After a year of herbal and dietary supplements, Tristan was active and healthy Growing at a normal rate, by age 5 he was in the 90 percentile for height and weight!

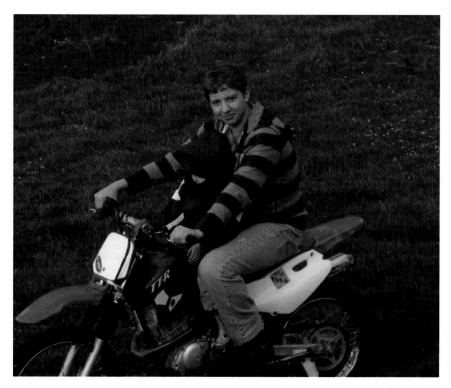

Tristan today, at 16 he loves the Montana outdoors and his little brother!

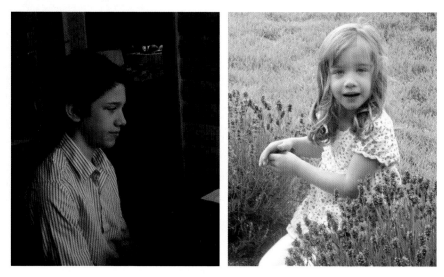

Brian and Heidi, our miracles after being told it was impossible for us to have more children.

What I did find to be helpful in preventing infections was **Parsley Tea** sweetened with a bit of honey, to which the contents of two **Cranberry** capsules were added for each one pint of tea. This was sipped throughout the day until the capsules could be swallowed. Later, I discovered **D-mannose,** available in freeze-dried Aloe Vera, Ambrotose Complex or ClearTract. This glyconutrient is thought to coat the inside of the bladder, thus preventing detrimental bacteria from adhering and causing infection. Recently, I have found **Golden Rod** extract to be helpful. With the help of these supplements, Tristan has been infection-free for up to two years at a time rather than being on prophylactic antibiotics as a preventative.

"KEEP DOING WHAT YOU ARE DOING, MAMA."

In this chapter, I have shared the simple herbs and supplements that I have found to be helpful in giving our son a normal life. I have done so to encourage others who face similar difficulties to also find answers and hope. Not all of these herbs have been under the microscope of rigorous scientific research and trials. However, beyond a shadow of doubt, they have given my son what dialysis could not—12 years of normal life and relatively good health. In the early years, his pediatrician was curious about how much of a difference was being made by what I was giving Tristan. To answer his questions, I agreed to discontinue all the herbs and supplements for six weeks and to bring my son in for blood work. The lab results showed a significant decrease in kidney function during this time. I will never forget his kind words to me, "Keep doing what you are doing, Mama. It is working and is more than I can do for him."

While we are still seeking for complete healing for Tristan, we have been blessed to beat the odds in so many ways. Seventy percent of little boys born with this condition die within the first two weeks of life, but our son survived for two years with the blockage in place. Children with severe kidney damage do not grow normally. At 16, Tristan is almost six feet tall, making him taller than Dad. We give thanks for every pain-free, healthy day he enjoys, and we confidently expect to find complete healing in the days ahead.

CHAPTER ELEVEN

ADRENAL AND THYROID GLANDS

THE ADRENAL GLANDS

The triangular-shaped adrenal glands are part of the endocrine system and sit at the top of the kidneys. They produce certain hormones and regulate mineral and water balance. When we are frightened or angered, they produce testosterone, enabling the muscles to do things we couldn't under normal circumstances. Chiefly responsible for the body's response to stress, the adrenal glands release cortisol, a type of steroid, whenever challenging situations are encountered.

The list of challenges for many of us is lengthy: lack of sleep, financial pressure, relationship turmoil, moving, and death or illness of a loved one, to name just a few. Cortisol release does its best to help us meet these challenges, but overstimulation caused by constant stress is destructive to the body and can result in adrenal exhaustion.

Symptoms of adrenal exhaustion can include the following:

- Feeling most energetic at night
- Consistently low blood pressure
- Intense sensitivity to cold
- Unable to cope with stress
- Slow recovery from illness or injury
- Waking up tired
- Constant exhaustion
- Weight gain
- Hair loss
- Arthritis
- Need coffee to get going in the morning
- Low libido

The good news is that herbs can help restore the adrenal glands, give you energy, and reduce your dependence on stimulants such as caffeine or nicotine. **Eleuthero,** formerly known as Siberian Ginseng, is perhaps the most widely used herb to support the adrenal glands. It prevents the excessive release of cortisol. **Codonopsis Root** has been used in China for more than 2,000 years. It is the best known and most widely used adaptogen. Adaptogens are substances that nonspecifically enhance and regulate the body's ability to withstand stress.

Astragulus and **Ashwagandha** are used to relieve fatigue. **Fo-Ti Root** is one of the top four most important Chinese herbs and is highly prized as an adaptogen. It is also used to restore hair loss and increase libido. **Wild Yam** contains compounds that are similar in structure to steroids, which provide the building blocks for complex glandular processes. Related to **Eleathero**, **Devil's Club** encourages weight loss and relieves arthritis. A liquid combination of these herbs, such **Adren- L-Aid,** along with a healthy diet and exercise can rejuvenate overworked adrenal glands.

Seven to nine hours of restful sleep is needed to maintain good health and is essential to restoring impaired adrenal function. Additional herbs can help when stress levels are high, especially if sleeping patterns are being disrupted. Throughout the day, a combination of **Catnip, Hops, Passionflower, St. John's Wort, Scullcap and Eleuthero** can be used to relax and calm the central nervous system, relieve anxiety, and support the body's ability to handle stress. With less stress build-up from the day, unwinding and falling asleep becomes much easier at bedtime. **Stress and Sleep**

When Bedtime Drops Are Helpful ...

During times of intense emotional stress, more support may be needed to get a good night's sleep. **Valerian Root** acts as a soother and depressor of the central nervous system. High in calcium, it has a very calming effect. **Hops** acts as a mild sedative and is often combined with Valerian. **Passionflower** relieves restlessness, irritability, and difficulty falling asleep. **Scullcap** contains sedative properties and is used to treat insomnia. Taking a liquid extract combination of these herbs, such as **Bedtime Drops**, twenty minutes before bedtime and repeating the dosage as needed could make the difference between a miserable night and a restful one.

Focus on eating plenty of fresh or lightly steamed vegetables and their juices to help restore your fatigued or exhausted adrenal glands. Fasting and detoxing should be avoided until you feel better. Add foods to your diet that are high in potassium, such as sunflower seeds, almonds, raisins and avocados. Avoid foods high in sodium and sugar and simple carbohydrates. Eating frequent, small light meals rather than large heavy ones is also a kindness to the adrenal glands. See Chapter Three for herbs to support the adrenal glands during pregnancy.

THE THYROID

Also part of the endocrine system, the thyroid is a small bow tie or butterfly-shaped gland. Located in the neck and wrapped around the windpipe, it sits behind and below the "Adam's Apple" area. The thyroid produces several hormones, of which two are key: triodothyronine (T3) and thyroxine (T4). These hormones help oxygen get into cells, and determine the body's basal metabolic rate. The thyroid is truly the master of metabolism. This little gland also contains the only cells in the body capable of absorbing the iodine needed to produce hormones.

Hypothyroidism, or an underactive thyroid, occurs most frequently in women over the age of 40; however, men and teenagers are not exempt. More prevalent than previously thought, hypothyroidism is believed to be affecting up to 10 percent of the population to some degree. Approximately 50 percent of those who suffer from subclinical hypothyroidism are unaware of the problem. The most observable sign is a low body temperature when awakening in the morning.

Other symptoms of an underactive thyroid can include the following:

- Weight gain
- Inability to lose weight
- Dry, brittle hair
- Hair loss
- Dry, gritty eyes
- Eye tics
- Feeling sluggish and tired
- Difficulty concentrating
- Becoming more forgetful
- Infertility
- Easy bruising
- Thin, brittle nails
- Feeling cold when others are comfortable

Except for **Guggul** extract and **Parsley** extract, the herbs most beneficial to the under active thyroid are much easier to ingest in capsule or tablet form. **Irish Moss** and **Kelp** are both excellent sources of electrolyte minerals and iodine, which are essential to normal thyroid function. In liquid extract form, these are extremely unpleasant with a stomach-turning odor. **Guggul** extract containing guggulsterones stimulates the production thyroid hormones and is not unpleasant in liquid form. **Parsley** is rich in trace and electrolyte minerals. While it does not contain iodine, it is frequently included in herbal combinations used to support the thyroid.

Since so much of the basal metabolic rate (rate at which energy is used by a body at complete rest) is controlled by the thyroid,

The thyroid is key to a healthy metabolic rate. it makes sense for individuals who are overweight and unable to lose pounds to support this little gland with appropriate supplements. Whenever impaired thyroid function is suspected, it is wise to avoid toothpaste and mouthwash that contain fluoride, as it may further slow down the thyroid. Soy milk was found by the University of Michigan to increase hypothyroidism and should also be avoided.

WINNING WITH WEIGHT CONTROL

A specific combination of herbs in a liquid extract can be very effective in helping the thyroid function normally and in supporting weight loss, especially for those who exercise regularly and have a reasonable diet but are still unable to shed unwanted pounds and inches. **Evodia** naturally suppresses the appetite. Brazilian **Porangaba Leaf** reduces the amount of food needed to feel full. **Garcinia Fruit** inhibits the conversion of dietary carbohydrates to fat and is most effective when taken three times daily. Recent research indicates that **Pomegranate Leaf** inhibits fat absorption in the intestinal tract.

Ginger and **Evodia** increase thermogenesis, the burning of calories to increase body temperature. A three-month double-blind, placebo-controlled trial found that administering a **Guggul**-based formula to overweight subjects resulted in the loss of 12.1–12.7 pounds compared to the placebo-receiving group. Malic acid, found in **Horsetail** and **Cornsilk,** is used by the Krebs cycle, the final and essential step in making energy from carbohydrates, fats, and protein available for use by the body.

Recently, a close friend dropped 30 pounds with this particular combination of herbs, **Weight Control Formula** available from Mountain Meadow Herbs. Previously, she had been unable to lose weight in spite of being an avid runner and eating a moderate diet.

Graves' disease is caused by an overactive thyroid and is less common than hypothyroidism. It is considered to be an autoimmune disease and occurs seven to ten times more frequently in women than in men.

Symptoms of Grave's disease can include:

- Weight loss
- Nervousness
- Sweating
- Goiter
- Protruding eye (called proptosis)

A doctor's diagnosis should be obtained when this condition is suspected. Aspartame is thought to contribute to Graves' disease and should be strictly avoided.

Bungle Weed may be used to alleviate an overactive thyroid. It contains inorganic acids which lower thyroxine and thyrotrophin levels in the body. **Balm** may help as well by inhibiting the attachment of the antibodies that cause Graves' disease to affect the thyroid gland. These herbs should be used under the supervision of a qualified care giver. Graves' is a serious disease, if left untreated, it can cause heart failure and death

CHAPTER TWELVE

THE MOUNTAIN
MEADOW HERBS
STORY

D estiny can be hidden inside the very thing we wish had never
come our way. Taking the lemon of Tristan's illness and
making lemonade has been an unbelievable journey of discovery
and fulfillment. Relieving suffering by creating natural remedies
that have benefited tens of thousands has brought me unspeakable
joy. If given the choice, I would, no doubt have chosen an easier path
to compassion. But in reality, difficulty created an environment for
the discovery of a gift I was unaware I had been given. Using the
talent I have been given has changed me dramatically as a person;
but more importantly, it has benefited many others, which is the
true reason for the gift.

By 2003, as friends and family heard of Tristan's remarkable
recovery and continued good health, requests for customized
solutions to meet similar health challenges were pouring in from
across the country. Since I was already making my own extracts

for him, at first, it was easy to do the research, order in the appropriate herbs, and create simple remedies to meet these needs. However, without intending to, I was building a business that needed to be organized. My wonderful entrepreneurial husband recognized long before I did that my hobby had huge potential. Nathan took it upon himself to convert the garage into a state-licensed facility where I could legally produce more of the golden extracts I had fallen in love with. I painted the walls a cheery yellow, and spent some of the happiest hours of my life researching, creating, and carefully packaging herbal formulations to relieve the suffering of others.

Discovering which herbs would bring relief to a specific condition and then creating a formulation became the favorite part of what I was doing. Breathless with excitement, I felt that each project was like going into another realm. Hours would go by, but it seemed as though only 15 minutes had passed instead of half a day. My brain shifted into a different mode as insights and connections were made. This was never exhausting and always energizing because I was doing exactly what I was created to do. When notes and phone calls confirmed my work, I often wept out of sheer joy, gratitude, and wonder at the opportunity I had been given.

As an Amish/Mennonite girl helping my parents on the farm, my dreams of being a nurse when I grew up consumed a large part of my younger years. Perhaps it was the comforting touch of the sweet-faced nurse who fed me ice cream and Jello after my tonsils were removed that sparked the desire. Or it may have been going with my mother through the dark night to bring our little friend to the nearest hospital in rural Costa Rica. This was a crowded, indifferent place, and the little girl I had held and played with lay strangely silent as she was returned to her weeping mother. I watched my mother sew a little white dress the next afternoon and was present at the tiny grave. At five years old, the big words like "pneumonia" swirling around me made no sense, but I began to understand suffering. My dream of being a registered nurse was never realized, but this dream was born out of a desire to ease suffering, and God has not forgotten.

This dream was born out of a desire to ease suffering, and God has not forgotten.

Midwives are an important and trusted part of Amish culture, and my mother-in-law was a caring and highly respected one for 26 years. Her faith in me and in natural healing gave me a lot of confidence in the early days as I searched for answers for our son. I was deeply honored in 2001 when, at a family Christmas gathering, she asked me to create herbal combinations to use in her large practice. As we worked together, I gave her my very best efforts. Over the next year and a half, various combinations were tested and perfected to make pregnancy, childbirth, and nursing a better experience for new moms under her care. These products went on to become our core line and contributed enormously to the success of Mountain Meadow Herbs.

OVERCOMING OBSTACLES

However, success did not come to me without difficulties that needed to be overcome. I was painfully shy with little more than an eighth-grade formal education. In the Amish culture, this is considered sufficient; however, in my early twenties, I studied and received a General Education Diploma (GED).

A condition known as "number dyslexia" made dialing phone numbers difficult and bookkeeping impossible. Because I was raised to be a wife and mother rather than a business woman, I experienced intense guilt and confusion as the enterprise grew. Once we were licensed and officially in business, I did a small amount of marketing, followed by an alarming number of orders. My husband and I found ourselves working late at night after our boys were asleep, filling orders, making extracts, bottling, and labeling products. To keep up with demand, Nathan designed new equipment including a large herb press, which made the process much easier. Growth required constant change, and processes needed to be documented to ensure quality was not lost as it became evident that the two of us were no longer able to keep up with demand.

First I hired a bookkeeper to compensate for my biggest weakness. Then we enlisted a young energetic friend who was initially hired to help with the household work that had been left undone for too long. Carolyn was smart and capable and able to do much more than housework. As fall approached, I found myself needing to choose between home-schooling Tristan and Brian and continuing to run the daily operations. I chose to follow my heart. After careful training, Carolyn proved completely trustworthy, and all but product-development and marketing were turned over to her care. Since lovely young ladies of her caliber do not go unnoticed, we lost her to a fine young gentleman from Canada in

September of 2005. By this time, she had accomplished her goal of "turning this all into a real business," as she was fond of saying.

Growth was also happening outside of Mountain Meadow Herbs. Little Heidi joined our family on July 23, 2005. After the devastating loss of a tiny son two years earlier, our hearts were healed as we held and cared for our new daughter. To me she was and still is tangible evidence of God's goodness. Six weeks after her birth, having outgrown its humble beginnings, Mountain Meadow Herbs was moved out of our home and into a new and much larger facility. By now, there were four full-time employees, and we were bursting at the seams.

A CULTURE OF CARING

I had not set out to build a big business. My goal had been to help sick people, but there were far too many requests for me to care for on my own. I feared that some person in need would be treated with indifference or in an uncaring manner by our employees. To avoid this, I based hiring criteria on the things I cared about most deeply, and being a caring person was definitely at the top of the list. Those who answered the phone were trained to remain on the line until they knew the person on the other end felt cared for and respected. Obviously, we knew we could not help everyone, but we could genuinely care. We also discovered that passing up professionals in favor of those who were eager to learn, had a great work ethic, and consistently treated others with kindness and respect made for an incredible team.

Treating our employees as we would want to be treated—with fairness, respect and care—created an unusual workplace environment. On more than one occasion I walked into the building to find two or more employees working after hours. They were quick to assure me that they had clocked out and had just forgotten to go home. Judging by the stack of orders, I knew the real reason for their lingering was to make sure packages were shipped within 24 hours because it was important to me that our customers received their orders quickly.

Several employees, including our amazing general manager, took significant pay cuts to come be a part of a caring family culture where they could grow as individuals. When one employee lost a daughter to cancer in another state, the hat was passed to help with travel expenses—and it was not my idea! The gifts and talents of each employee were valued and respected by placing them in positions within the company where they could flourish. Leading and working with this team that eventually grew to 16 special people was truly an honor, and their loyalty and affection were priceless.

Creating products that make a difference has always been very important to me. Perhaps it was the desperation of my son's condition that made it impossible for me to offer a product lightly to customers who trusted our company and the brand we were creating. In any case, opportunities to market the latest and greatest new product to our growing clientele came across my desk regularly. I chose, instead, to offer only products I truly believed in and would use myself or give to my children. At Mountain

Meadow Herbs, compromising integrity to create a profit was, and is today, unacceptable and a breach of customer trust.

GROWING FROM THE HEART

In those early days, I led our fledgling company largely from my heart. Growing from serving fewer than 100 customers to more than 25,000 in five short years was exhilarating and scary. I lived through times of sheer panic. My father was a brilliant dairy farmer and example for me. His attention to detail, willingness to get rid of what was not working, and common sense had led to profitability during times when others were exiting farming in masses and blaming their demise on low milk prices. I turned to these lessons, books, mentors and my faith to compensate for lack of education in business. Certain books such as *The E-Myth* would keep coming up in conversations or articles until I would notice, get the book, and read it. Without fail, the answer to an issue I was facing was hidden in its pages.

My earliest mentor was a wise woman whom I greatly loved and respected. At our first meeting, I was complaining, and she was very direct in instructing me to go back to work and do with joy what was in front of me to do. Her wisdom also led me to pray for a business mentor or coach rather than to pursue education in business. The answer came in the form of Dr. Lance Wallnau, whose coaching and friendship through the years has been priceless.

Nathan's belief in me and what we were doing was the greatest gift in those years. He was also the one who set goals and inspired us all. In September of 2006, I knew we needed to do something different in order to reach our year-end goal. We were stuck, and the team celebration we all were looking forward to was slipping away. During this time, an email from a missionary friend in India caught my eye. As I read of the suffering and need there, I was impressed to give $5,000 to cover the cost of a meeting to encourage leaders.

Cash was scarce, and I dreaded telling both our general manager, who did all the purchasing, and our bookkeeper to send a check in this amount to India. However, Nathan was in agreement, and both girls were gracious in spite of their fear. With prayer for joy among the persecuted church to be the result of our gift, the check was mailed. We broke through our ceiling the next month with more than enough money to pay the bills. Then a grateful email came filled with the details of deeper joy and love as believers came together in India. These beautiful people spent an entire afternoon thanking God for our generosity and praying for blessing on Mountain Meadow Herbs! Apparently heaven heard. We went on to exceed our year-end goal and celebrated grandly.

MISTAKES ARE PART OF THE STORY TOO

Although I have been blessed with wonderful mentors, books, and unbelievable favor, I have also made some serious mistakes. The worst ones cost me a part of the Mountain Meadow Herbs family and led to having to make a painful but unavoidable decision. In 2007, I made two grave errors at the same time. I was expecting our third child within a few months when my marketing assistant, realizing she would not be able to take on marketing and school at the same time, resigned. At the same time, we had outgrown the software used for all data, including bookkeeping.

Knowing little about software, I took the easiest route and told our general manager and bookkeeper to handle this problem. Also, pressured by the soon-coming baby, I hired the first person to respond to my desperate advertisement for help in marketing.

Both decisions ended up as disasters. The new software was worse than a nightmare, sold by a company with little integrity. The marketing expert I hired cost us an unmentionable figure and offended our customers. No profit and loss statements could be extracted from the new software, and all this was happening while I was busy with a newborn. Three months of serious losses accrued without us knowing there was a problem.

Faced with either letting employees go or losing the business, I knew what had to be done. I based my decisions on our core values, keeping those employees who most consistently lived our values and were able to work efficiently and effectively in more than one department. Over the next five months, the company returned to profitability, but I deeply grieved the loss of five workers.

I based my decisions on our core values.

GRATEFUL BEYOND WORDS

Soft Christmas music greeted me along with the smiling faces of precious friends as I walked into the room carrying our three-month-old son. White tablecloths topped with deep red poinsettias and flickering candles covered the round tables. Little girls in festive dresses twirled around the room. Boys, dressed in their best, chased each other as fast as they dared. The smell of holiday delicacies promised that a delicious meal was waiting. We were here to celebrate another year of God's goodness, the privilege of working together, and the honor of creating and providing natural health solutions to relieve suffering.

Sitting with my husband and children, my eyes lingered on the face of our oldest son, Tristan. From the ashes of despair, beauty had been created, and my heart was overwhelmed. The evening was magical. Speeches were made; some brought tears, and others were so funny we couldn't stop laughing. United in making a difference through genuine caring and natural health solutions, these were among my dearest friends, and I loved each one deeply. Bonuses were handed out, and each employee was given an award, not based on performance but on the value they brought to the company and what we loved about each one. Like a little bit of heaven, liquid love filled the room. Father God was with us, and He was the true reason for all we had been given.

CHAPTER THIRTEEN
MALARIA: THE NEXT CHALLENGE

Every 30 seconds, a child dies from malaria. As we enjoyed dinner tonight, 120 mothers were left to grieve the loss of a son or daughter who died needlessly from a mosquito bite. Malaria was largely eradicated from developed countries by the early seventies through the use of insecticides and drugs. Unfortunately, efforts to wipe out the disease on a global scale slacked off as market demand decreased and resistance to the drugs and insecticides grew.

In the past decade, increased funding and awareness have grown with the help of The Bill and Melinda Gates Foundation and Malaria No More. Their support has made an impressive difference through nets, drugs and targeted spraying. In some areas, deaths from malaria have decreased by 40 to 80 percent. Despite these advances, the problem remains huge, and there is a lot left to be done, particularly in Africa and South America.

Typically, drugs used to treat malaria are derived from the Wormwood herb and then combined with an antibiotic to increase effectiveness. The more I learned, the more curious I became to find out if the correct combination of herbal extracts would do the same thing. So, with the help of my production manager, research was done and a formula created to kill the protozoa. A second combination was developed to heal the liver damage caused by malaria and to help the body recover fully. Anticipation ran high in the summer of 2007, as 24 bottles of what we hoped to be life-saving liquid was shipped to Bozeman, Montana, and then on to Uganda.

Forms to document the results of the formulas were included in the shipment bound for a Uganda Orphans' Fund clinic in the Kasozi village of Uganda. A few months later, I received a short but very welcome email stating that the herbs were working within 24 hours, even in severe cases! The forms were not returned, but having lived in a third-world country, I understood. I also realized a much more hands-on approach and strong relationships would be needed to establish the value of the herbs and their results. Because I was expecting our fourth child at this point, I knew this was not the right time for me to pursue this matter.

The herbs were working—even in severe cases!

However, causes of poverty and disease have interested me for many years, and I hope to one day make a significant contribution in this area. While the success of Mountain Meadow Herbs enabled us to give financially into organizations that are making a difference, the longing for more hands-on involvement refuses to be stilled. Even the eventual funding of an orphanage and providing food and clothes for 120 orphans left me slightly dissatisfied. One day in April of 2008, I found myself praying, "God, if it is time to move on, please bring a buyer for this business. I have no idea how to find one, and since we are hidden away in Montana, I'll know it's really You if one shows up."

Two weeks later, I was shocked to receive a letter from a broker in Kansas City, Missouri, informing me that a naturopathic doctor from Switzerland wanted to buy an herbal company. Since ours fit his criteria, would we be interested in selling? For two weeks, I carried the letter in my work bag before sharing it with anyone, and I struggled with letting go in order to create space for the future. Both Nathan and I felt the time was right, and six months later, my time as the mother of Mountain Meadow Herbs and its team ended. At our favorite restaurant, I thanked the team over dinner for the honor of leading them. We ate, laughed, and cried far into the night.

The surprises did not end with the sale of the company. As I came to know the new owner, I discovered we share a common interest in malaria. I learned that a professor in Seattle had discovered a portion of the malaria protozoa is magnetic in structure and can be manipulated and killed with magnetic fields. Since no part of the human body is magnetic, this is a safe and exciting new technology. My new friend went on to develop a prototype to apply this technology and tested it with impressive results in Ghana, Africa. Professors in Kenya, Africa, are on board to conduct clinical trials to scientifically document and establish this as an effective malaria treatment.

The combination of using magnetic fields and herbal extracts to kill malaria protozoa presents options worth pursuing in ending death from malaria once and for all. Wormwood can be grown with little water, and the tree whose bark provides quinine is grown in the Congo. Could it be possible that a simple tea made from plants that naturally grow where they are needed most could be as effective as the extracts sent to Uganda in 2007? If this is the case, the problem becomes much easier, with no need for equipment and all that is involved in making extracts. These and many other questions are ones I hope find answers to next. Ultimately a way must be found for even the remotest village to cure and heal its children and adults from malaria.

Since 2007 another third world clinic, missionaries and Wycliffe bible translators have tired the herbal extracts for malaria. Feedback has been sparse but what has come in has been positive. A missionary friend, who lost her young son to cerebral malaria in 2011, contacted me to explore the possibility of using herbal extracts as a prophylactic to protect against contracting malaria. A simple blend of **Wormwood, Green tea** and **Propolis resin** extracts, **Malair-Shield** was made and sent to the grieving missionary family who reported that it seemed to be working after using it for a month during the rainy season, no one had contracted malaria.

The three formulas for malaria went on to become part of the line of Mountain Meadow Herbs products available to anyone interested in trying them for foreign travel or longer stays in malaria prone areas. Malaria is a serious illness, please keep in mind that there are no clinical trials or FDA approval for using these herbal combinations to prevent, treat or cure this disease. This is particularly important to keep in mind in determining when to seek conventional medical intervention while abroad.

The Malair-Sheild is most popular with families who spend extended time in foreign countries. The drugs used to prevent malaria are very hard on the liver, can cause upset stomach, anxiety, exacerbate skin problem, and should not be used by nursing or pregnant women. Unfortunately, the areas that are sensitive to the long standing use of Melfloquine and Floroquine as a malaria prophalytic are shrinking. The parasite is a complex organism, that avoids the immune system by constantly changing it's surface. The Center Of Disease Control lists Melarone, a newer drug, as the first protective option for foreign travel to the many areas that are now resistant. Melarone contains two active ingredients, proguanil hydrochloride and atovaquone that work to stop the parasite in the blood from reproducing which leads to the disease.

The artemisia compounds in Wormwood work by concentrating in the parasite infected red blood corpruscles where they are thought to create free radical damage to parasite membranes. The parasite is then phagocytosed or ingested and cleared by white blood cells. Long term use as a preventative is controversial, the more conservative resources such as the PRD for Herbal Medicines caution against long term use due to its thujone content causing mental disturbances when used continuously. Large amounts can lead to vomiting, dizziness, headaches and disturbances of the central nervous system and miscarriage.

Thujone is present in other common plants that when used in moderation, have no know side effects. These include sage, oregano, cypress, junipers, yarrow and mint. A toxicity study on mice found the lethal dose of thujone to be around 45mg/kg. The compound was discovered after absinthe, a high volume alcohol spirit, became popular in the mid 19th century. Originating in Switzerland, it contains fennel, anise and other herbs and went on to become very popular among the Parisian writers and artists. Because of its connection to the Bohemian culture, conservatives strongly opposed its use.

Dr. Valentin Magnan, who studied alcoholism, tested pure wormwood oil on animals and discovered it caused seizures independent from the effects of alcohol. Based on this, it was assumed that absinthe, which contains a small amount of wormwood oil, was more dangerous than ordinary alcohol. Eventually thujone was isolated as the cause of these reactions. Magnan went on to study 250 abusers of alcohol and noted that those who drank absinthe had seizures and hallucinations. In light of modern evidence, these conclusions are questionable, as they are based on a poor understanding of other compounds and diseases, and clouded by Magnan's belief that alcohol and absinthe were "degenerating" the French race and its sale in Europe was banded.

Only recently have the studies and beliefs about thujone been questioned and further researched. While it's molecular structure was found to be similar to the active compound found in cannabis that is responsible for its mind altering effect, a 1999 study proved the assumption of thujone having a similar effect to be false. It is also important to note that many of the studies done on thujone used the essential oil wormwood in the study. Wormwood oil naturally contains a higher concentration of thujone and other active compounds than a wormwood extract, tea or capsule. For those who are faced with needing to choose a way to prevent or treat malaria, my best advice is to learn everything you can about the modern medical options and those offered by nature, then go with what you are comfortable with.

In addition to Wormwood , the dried bark of 6-8 year old Cinchona trees is a very valuable malaria treatment. Also known as quinine for at least 300 years, it interferes with the parasites ability to reproduce its self. Combining an extract of this bark with Wormwood and extracts that have a strong, natural antibiotic effect such as **Olive** leaf and **Propolis** resin extract, creates a powerful natural anti-malarial. Anti-oxidants are thought to increase Wormwoods effect on the parasites; I chose my favorites, **Bilberry** and **Green tea** to complete the formula now known as **Malair-X.**

Recovering from a serious bout of malaria can be long and difficult, taking weeks or months. When the parasite arrives in the human body via a mosquito bite it heads for the liver. Here it changes into a new form to avoid the immune system that also allows it to invade red blood cells. The parasite reproduces in the liver cells, the cells burst open releasing thousands of parasites into the bloodstream where they infect more red bloods cells and the cycle is repeated. The bursting cells are responsible for the fever and chills that come with malaria. The liver enlarges as does the spleen in the course of the disease. Other major organs that can be damaged are the kidneys and the brain. Feeling weak and depleted for months is common when recovering from malaria.

Herbs have a long history of helping the body heal, and can be big help in a full return to vibrant health. **Astragalus** can help with the fatigue and has gentle healing effect . Bitter herbs are the liver best friend, **Quassia** bark extract is a great choice to encourage healthy liver function. Red blood cell loss no doubt contributes to the weakness experienced in the recovery phase. As a tonic for the immune system, **Echinacea** may increase red and white blood cell count and improve their function. It is valuable in the recovery of many viral and bacterial diseases. The malaria parasite can continue to lie dormant in the liver for up to 4 years, **Neem** and **Pau D Arco** may be helpful in preventing a relapse during the recovery by suppressing the parasite and preventing reproduction. **Chamomile** can help soothe the inflammation of the major organs affected by the disease and help calm the central nervous system. A combination of these or similar herbs can be taken for 3-6 months to help the body heal and fully recover. **Malair-Mend**

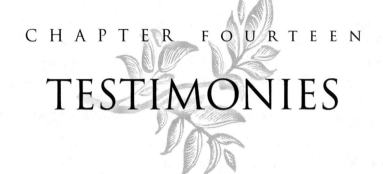

CHAPTER FOURTEEN

TESTIMONIES

GENERAL

Greetings across the miles … Just thought I'd take this time to Thank You for your ever ready service, your support and prayer along with your beneficial products that offer hope and health to those who receive them. Mountain Meadow Herbs has been like an answered prayer in my life. Of all the places I've dealt with, I always come back to you as the best. While there are many out there with good products, my formed impression (whether right or wrong!) is that while their products keep a healthy person in good health, yours help an unhealthy person to good health. May God's blessings be with you and may He be glorified for sending health and hope through people like you! I'm getting good results with the Yeast X and hope to do the Adren-L-Aid in a few months. As long as Mountain Meadow Herbs exists, you'll find me as one of your satisfied and happy customers.

*–*LINDA L.

CHILDBIRTH

I bought Gentle Birth Formula from you earlier this spring/summer. We had our 2nd baby born to us in July. I did not use the Gentle Birth with our 1st one and had a long / hard labor and the pain was HORRIBLE! I took it with our 2nd one and what a difference! I had no pain once I was 10 centimeters, and the Dr. couldn't believe the difference. We had a healthy girl weighing 8lbs 4oz, and my Dr. couldn't believe I had her without an epidural. What a good feeling. I would not dread having to go thru labor again with Gentle Birth. Just want to thank you and would recommend this product to anyone.

—MRS. BRICKER

I just had my 8th baby yesterday. I purchased Gentle Birth Formula because I did not want to have another 20 hr labor. My average is about 16 hrs. I was a little skeptical at first, but willing to give this a try. When I received the product, I only had 4 wks till my due date. As it turned out, I only used it for about 3 wks since my little guy came early. I woke up with contractions at 1:30. They were coming every 3-4 min. Three hours later, my baby was born. I was shocked at how fast it went. I also am bleeding so much less this time around. My midwife was even surprised at how little blood I lost afterwards. I feel great and am so happy that I found this product. I know God had His hand in it, but I believe Gentle Birth Formula helped tremendously.

—JILL

I've had three home births, each as smooth and manageable as can be imagined. The tincture made contractions very effective and productive without being excruciating, consistently five minutes apart throughout the entirety of my labors. Recovery was short; I stopped bleeding within the first week. Highly recommend.

—ERIN

I had a C-section with my first baby because of failing to progress. The next two were about the same, laboring for 18 hours then being induced and drugged, both successful VBACs but obviously long and interfered with. I took Gentle Birth Formula from 37 weeks until my due date during my fourth pregnancy. Three days after my due date mild contractions began. I relaxed in a tub of warm water, and then it was really time to go. As we arrived at the hospital, I was surprised to feel the head crowning already. We left the car running with the doors open at the front of the hospital. Lying on the bed a few minutes later and with no interference of drugs or needles, I gracefully delivered my 9 lb 12 oz little boy! I was so stunned that my labor and delivery were all done. I give a lot of thanks and praise for this product, and I tell everyone I know.

—DEBBIE MARTENS

The Gentle Birth Formula prolonged my labor long enough for my midwife to get here! I usually go so fast, she doesn't have enough time. You said in your brochure that it helped with longer labors for those who usually have precipitated births, and that was definitely the case with me.

—MRS. HOUSER

I just wanted to sing the praises of Gentle Birth Formula! With my first child, I had to be induced a week late and the labor was long (14 hours), horrendously painful, and absolutely NOT the birth experience I wanted! I had to get three epidurals, which I really didn't want, and push for almost 2 hours to deliver a 6 lb., 11 oz. girl. When I was pregnant with my second child, I discovered Gentle Birth and began taking it at 36 weeks (a little late, even!). I ended up going into labor 5 days early & the whole birthing process (from waking up with contractions 5 minutes apart to delivering) was less than 6 hours.

We were only in the hospital for an hour & a half before the baby was born! I was able to deliver with NO pain medication and pushed for approximately 10 minutes to deliver an 8 lb., 12 oz. baby boy! It was amazing and exactly what I'd hoped my birth would be. I credit Gentle Birth with helping me have the drug-free, fast delivery that I'd always hoped for! Thank you so much!!

—CATHERINE

I did not know I was in labor until I was in transition. From the time I had my first hard contraction till delivery was 1/2 hour! I couldn't believe it! I nearly beat the midwife by 5 min.! And my son was born with two pushes! My last two sons were also born with two pushes but with this one, the water bag popped as his head was being born.

—CLARA

One mother with her 1st baby had to be taken to the hospital where they gave her strong medication. She finally did have her baby. Now for her 2nd one, I gave her the Gentle Birth Formula. She was in labor only 4 hrs and had a nice delivery. She didn't bleed much and felt stronger after delivery. I really do recommend this product!

—MRS. GINGERICH (MIDWIFE)

Thank you for the fine products. I am pleased with the results: smooth, fast births especially 1st timers. Please don't compromise on quality!

—MRS. PETERSHEIM (MIDWIFE)

I have had some very nice births with Gentle Birth Formula. I've had mothers who used your product faithfully and said they can't believe it. It was so easy, and they felt so different. One 1st timer broke her water at 7am and had her baby at 10am and seemed very good.

—MRS. BONTRAGER (MIDWIFE)

Just a note to tell you I'm very impressed with the Gentle Birth Formula! I knew I was in labor all day, but contractions were very light. I did the cleaning and hung wash out on the line. Around 3'o clock, I was getting certain this was real labor and felt like resting. I called the midwife (my mom) at 3:30 and said I'd like if she'd come awhile, but felt silly — because surely this was just the beginning! Contractions were hard working ones by 4:00 and baby was born at 5:00, no complications. I had very little bleeding in the following weeks, less than for the first three babies. Many thanks for a great product!

—LORENE

I tried your Gentle Birth Formula after having tried many other things in that line, always to no avail. I was always overdue a few weeks, and a few times my labor had to be started with IV, which is all I expected for this time, with my 11th child. But I was in for a good surprise when at only 3 days overdue, I went into a quick labor and in a few hours had my baby. Praise the lord for every good thing, and thank you for a good product!

—SATISFIED IN PA

For my 9th child, I used the Gentle Birth Formula for the first time. I was in labor only 4 1/2 hrs and had only one push and she was born. I would recommend it to everybody! My labor was so much easier than the last two I had. I think I want another one!

—MRS. MILLER

The Gentle Birth Formula continues to be a loved formula by the mothers and their midwife (me). Thank you so much.

—EMMA

I received a call from a mother in labor who wanted to wait until contractions were more serious. Shortly afterwards the call came, asking me to come immediately. Driving as quickly as I could, to my dismay I was pulled over by a policeman. Ten minutes later, while trying convince the officer that I was on an important mission, my cell phone rang and a healthy baby boy was crying in the background. This was enough to validate my story, and I was not given a ticket. This mother had taken the Gentle Birth Formula and apparently did not experience the "serious" contractions she expected until the last twenty minutes before giving birth.

—MRS. COBLENTZ (MIDWIFE)

I just want to tell you what great products you handle. I had one miscarriage and the second time I started bleeding again, so I looked through the MMH book. I saw the C&B Formula, so we got a 4 oz. bottle. I took that for six hours and the bleeding completely stopped. I would never want to be without the C&B Formula during pregnancy. Thank you so much.

—E.Y.

NURSING

I was concerned with not having enough breast milk stashed when I returned to work and expressed this to my midwife. She asked me to try this product (Maxi-Milk) and told me to pump after every nursing session. What a relief to return to work knowing I had enough milk stocked for my baby! This product also helped me get my supply back up when I had a case of clogged ducts. After the initial resting period that the breast goes through to heal itself, my supply was back to normal with the help of the herbs in this supplement. Recommended to pregnant friends and a definite product to keep on hand for nursing moms!

—MARIA

I sure love your Maxi-Milk. For our first child, I could only nurse about a half of a year. Then, with our second child, my sister in law told me about the Maxi-Milk, so I decided to try it once. And now I can nurse her for over a year already.

—MRS. GINGERICH

If not for Maxi-Milk, I would have to give my babies bottles at a very young age. I don't have to give bottles at all! Its great!

—MATTIE

I love your Maxi-Milk. It keeps the little one satisfied and happy. I recommend it to everyone concerned with not having enough milk.

—MRS. HOSTETLER

Every time I get under stress or my supply is less, I can use Maxi-Milk and get good results. I don't want to be without it while nursing.

—LYDIA

We have 8 children and ALL of them I had to give bottles or else fed them soft foods quite young, which made fussy and constipated babies. With my last two, I used Maxi-Milk faithfully and with great results. I don't think I had more milk, but was more nourishing, and I had a satisfied and content baby.

—CLARA

When my daughter was 3 - 4 months old, I thought I needed to quit nursing, as I didn't have much milk for her. I used the Maxi-Milk, and within a couple days I saw a difference, so I used it for a couple of months and had lots of milk.

—BARBERA

This is my seventh baby. In the past I have never had very much milk, and my babies did not gain well. I decided I would give Maxi-Milk a good try. I now have more than enough milk and my baby is so chubby and happy! I actually cut back on the amount I was taking as my little girl was gaining 11 ounces per week.

—MRS. GINGERICH

I was struggling to meet the nursing needs of my 2-month-old twins. After a couple of days on Maxi-Milk, I could tell a difference. I was full and leaking milk! No more bottles, I was able to totally nurse them till they were over a year. Thanks for a great product!

—BARBARA

I've never had enough milk for my babies and I am so thankful for your Maxi-Milk. It's wonderful and so handy! I'm ordering more for myself and my sister-in-law so she can use it as well. Sometimes, I don't even take it every day, works wonderful!

—MRS. BORNTREGER

Thanks for sending me the Maxi-Milk. I could not breast feed my other three babies. Now this new one is very content, but she was fussy until I started taking Maxi-Milk! Now is very content and gaining well. Also, the Infant Tummy Aid has helped her stomach. I enjoy nursing now that she is content.

—MRS. FREY

Just a note to tell you how much I like Maxi-Milk! It worked for me the first day I started taking only 1/3 of the dose. I went from not having enough to having too much! Also my son was in a farm accident and spent four days in the hospital. My milk supply went down because of the stress and little sleep (I forgot my Maxi-Milk). As soon as I started taking it my milk supply was right back, even though I was still dealing with stress and lack of sleep! I don't know what I would have done without Maxi-Milk! Thank you so much for your wonderful products! May God richly bless.

—Karen H

I just want to share my testimony about your Maxi-Milk Tincture. When my little girl was two and a half weeks old, my milk was gone. (This is my first child) I never experienced any engorement or anything close to it. Everyone kept telling me my milk would eventually come in. Now I wish I would have ordered Maxi-Milk right away, but "live and learn!" Anyway, by this time she was just starving and crying all the time. I finally gave her some goat's milk and ordered Maxi-Milk. I didn't know if it was too late to get my milk in or not, but I wanted to try it because I REALLY wanted to nurse her. I had done a lot of reading on the benefits of mama's milk over formula. Anyway after taking the Maxi-Milk, I started having milk!!! I was soooo happy!! It was increasing in amount little by little every day. Again I never was engorged but I was nursing my baby!!!! I still have to supplement with goat milk, but she much prefers me over the bottle. I tried different ways of taking it, but what works best for me is to take a fairly large dose just before bedtime and I have the most milk that way. She is about 8 months old now and is still nursing. She is a happy baby and weighs 18 pounds! Come to find out, my mother and grandmother never could nurse their babies because of lack of milk. It really didn't matter to them because the bottle was the big thing back then. But I am so glad to be able to nurse mine!! Thank you, Thank you, Thank you!!!!

—Katherine

I wouldn't be nursing if I didn't have Maxi-Milk!"

—Mrs. Mast

"The Maxi-Milk is helping me so much. This product has been such a gift, as I have struggled with having the supply to meet the needs of my little one, especially after returning to work full time. It is allowing me to exclusively breast feed him."

—EMILY

Maxi-Milk, I need it ASAP, I love it! Now I have enough milk!

—BARBARA

"Please rush me another bottle of Maxi-Milk. Mine is getting low, and I don't want to run out cuz it is helping me after I tried many other products. So, thanks to the Maxi-Milk Formula!

—WILMA

I got some of your Maxi-Milk from my midwife and am very pleased with the results. It works! Now, I would like another bottle.

—DOROTHY

Thanks for the Christmas gifts. I use the planner to write my expected births in. Mothers are finding the Maxi-Milk makes for a more contented baby. It is really catching on.

—MRS. EICHER (MIDWIFE)

This is wonderful stuff! I am thoroughly enjoying nursing my 4th baby. I don't even have to worry about not having enough milk! I ran out of Maxi-Milk three days ago, and I can't wait to get more. I can tell my supply is not very plentiful. Is there anything like paying extra to have it shipped sooner? Thank you so much for your fantastic products! I have been recommending you to lots of my friends! Also, we have a specialty and bulk foods store and often get requests for teas or supplements for nursing mothers. Is there some way we could carry your products in our store? I would love to talk with someone about wholesale possibilities. Thank you again and God bless you all for using your talents to bring health to others!

—MRS. EBERSOLE

NEWBORNS

My mom gave me a bottle of your Herbal Calcium for our 3-yr-old son. He was very, very fussy as a baby, and he's never grown out of it. I started giving him that calcium and his crying spells have completely stopped. Often in the morning he'd cry for 1 1/2 hrs straight, and there was nothing I could do about it. Thanks for a Great Product!!

—MRS. RABER

I ordered this product because my 3-month-old son had a yeast diaper rash for 1 1/2 months that wouldn't go away even with prescription cream. I put the Olive Leaf Extract on his rash, and it was gone with in 48 hours.

—MEREDITH

Infant Tummy-Aid is our favorite product - when my son had colic this was like liquid gold to us - we tell every new parent about it!

—ABBY

The Infant Tummy-Aid works wonders for our 3-week-old son! I was nervous to use it at first, but at 2 weeks old, I'd rather try that than anything else. I'm glad I did! It had an instant calming effect for him!

—S. COOPER

LEG CRAMPS, TEETHING, BACKACHE, BLOOD PRESSURE

I love MMH products. Have not had any leg/foot cramps since about a week after starting the Herbal Calcium. I am 59 years old and was in the ER in April for excessively high blood pressure. Subsequent test showed off-the-charts cholesterol levels. In 4 months, with the herbal extracts and a couple of other supplements that target my issues, my results have been dramatic. I am thankful for those people who take the time to research and care for the health of others.

—JOY

Herbal Calcium is … great for babies who are teething. Makes happy babies and happy Moms!!

—MRS. E

I love the Herbal Calcium, I can't be without it while pregnant or I get cramps, foot spasms and tired, lower back and much more.

—MRS. MILLER

I take the Herbal Calcium during pregnancy, and I always sleep like a baby. I don't suffer from painful cramps, and it is wonderful to know it is a good calcium my body can use. I give it to my teething babies and also to my children when they complain of pain in their legs.

—HEIDI

I had back surgery this summer, after which I took Allevi-Rits with a Calcium supplement. After trying your Herbal Calcium, it really worked better and helped my back relax. The surgery didn't take all my pain away, as I have a curved back. When I am on my feet all day, I can feel the pain. When I take the two formulas together it improves by 75-80%.

—MRS. ZOOK

My mom gave me a bottle of your Herbal Calcium for our 3-year-old. He was very, very fussy as a baby and he's never grown out of it. I started giving him that calcium, and his crying spells have completely stopped. Often in the morning, he'd cry for 1 1/2 hrs straight, and there was nothing I could do about it. Thanks for a Great Product!!

—MRS.RABER

The Herbal Calcium has really helped my daughter while she's teething.

—N MILLER

Baby Karalyn started teething at 4 1/2 months. She was fussy, drooled a lot, and could hardly chew her fist and me hard enough! I started her on the Herbal Calcium and soon noticed a difference. Although it didn't totally eliminate her fussiness, she was more relaxed, quit chewing, and drooling! She gets all excited about the dropper bottles and opens her mouth for her "medicine". I gave some to my sister for her baby, and she's saying the same thing!

—MRS. COBLENTZ

The Herbal Calcium works wonderful! I'm using it on my 4 1/2 month old baby for teething and I'm almost out of it!

—MRS. KAUFFMAN

Please send us the Herbal Calcium immediately, as we're going on a trip and I'd really like to have it before then. I hate to be without it. It really helps me!

—ADA

Thank you for your prompt shipment of the Herbal Calcium. The last few nights, my daughter has slept a lot better.

—MRS. YODER

Here is an order for an 8-ounce Herbal Calcium. We have used one bottle for our 4-year-old twins and it has helped to keep them more calm and sleep better. Thank you. You have good products.

—MARTHA

I sure like the Herbal Calcium as I have such good results with it. I am almost 7 months pregnant and have had hardly any backache, which is new for me! With my other pregnancies I also used calcium (other kinds) and was still very much bothered with backache. So I give your calcium good credit. Thanks for making it available!

—MRS. YUTZY

I would like to order one 4 oz bottle of your Herbal Calcium. This is my 5th pregnancy and the first time I've gotten up to the 7th and 8th months without getting severe leg cramps, for which I am giving your calcium the credit.

—MRS. YODER

AFTER-PAINS, MENSTRUAL CRAMPS

I have 3 teenage daughters, and they and I benefit greatly from the Herbal Calcium effects when they have monthly cramps and discomfort. It works very quickly, and we go through lots of bottles. Thank you for a great product.

—ASHLEY R.

I like After-Pain Relief formula. If I have cramps, it just takes one does and its gone.

—EFFIE

My Favorite product is After-Pain Relief! I love this product. I take it directly under my tongue every 15 minutes. It does wonders. Not taking nearly as many pain pills. My after-pains are worse than my actual labor pains, so I was thrilled for this great product!

—WANDA

This herbal combination is wonderful. I started taking this After-Pain Relief as soon as my daughter was born and every time I nursed. I couldn't believe how it kept my cramping at a minimum, and my bleeding was considerable lighter. Thanks for such a wonderful product.

—MRS. PAULUS

I used your After-Pain Relief with baby number five. For the first time I was not counting hours until I could take more pain pills. I was very impressed!

—REGINA

Your After-Pain relief is wonderful! I normally have severe after-pains, but this time, it's been so nice to nurse my newborn without those dreaded pains!

—RELIEVED IN OH

I took the After-pain Relief every 15 minutes. It helped a lot! Usually I have a week to a week and a half of after-pains, but this time only two days!

—MRS. ZOOK

I used the Stomach Aid, Gentle Birth Formula, and After-Pain Relief. They really work! - Ruth

The After-Pain Relief has done wonders for my menstrual cramps that over-the-counter pain reliever didn't touch! I've recommended it to a few others with the same problems!

—J. YODER

Our daughters use the After-Pain Relief for their monthly and are almost completely pain free! Our oldest daughter used to get quite sick on the first day. My niece also uses it with the same results with more of their friends wanting to try it.

—MARY LOU

Just a few lines to let you know that I had a lot easier period this time, and I'm hoping it will keep on improving with more of your HB Formula and T&C Formula. I was having so much pain with my periods that I didn't do much all day long as I would just cramp and pain so much. Thanks again!

—MIRIAM

I am taking the T&C, and I think that I have ovulated tor the first time since my miscarriage! I can feel my period coming on, but it's not the painful, heavy flow like it always was. Thank you!

—TERESA

ACNE, IRREGULAR CYCLES

I just wanted to say thank you to you all. Several months back, all my periods were 2 weeks apart, so my mom got your HB and T&C Formulas. They REALLY worked!!! All my periods are back to normal, and I have no cramping. Before,I endured HORRIBLE cramps! Once again, thank you so much.

—K.R.R.

I started taking T&C on October 1st and I had an Ultrasound on November 1st, and the cyst and fibroids I had were gone!

—REGINA

I have been taking the HB & T&C for a year now. I love it. I had fibroid cyst and I feel so much better with less pain.

—LENA

I am amazed at how well the T&C, HB & Progesterone Cream, used as you suggested, have changed my life. No more painful and very long periods. My ovarian cyst has disappeared, and my cycle is like clockwork! My Doctor suggested surgery, but now that is no longer necessary. It has only been about 3 months, but what a difference! I feel like myself again! Thank you so much.

—HOLLY

I really love the HB Formula. I used to have my cycle every two weeks, but this keeps me regular and helps a lot with my acne!

—M. GRABER

HB Formula works so well for my acne. I am very pleased!"

—RHONDA

My daughter usually had her periods late and got awful migraines. She decided to try your HB Formula, and it works wonderful! Her periods are on time, and she has only had two very slight migraines. "I want more; I hate to be without it!"

—MRS. LAPP

After using your products, I got my period. I have not had it for 2 years! The T&C and the HB Formula worked in just a little over a month. Thank you so much!

—AMANDA

I tried T&C and HB Formula to get my hormones regulated and to feel better. Within one month I was pregnant after trying for 6 years and having two miscarriages!

—MRS. GRAYBILL

Your HB Formula is working very well for our daughter who used to be so irregular.

—MRS. CHRISTNER

I was having my period every 13 days and after taking the HB Formula for one month, my cycle is every 32 days. I am impressed!!!

—CINDY

PMS, BABY BLUES

Head Ease lives up to its name! I had been experiencing migraine headaches for some time. I desired a product to help me "reset" whatever was "off" in my system(s). The first time I took Head Ease, at the beginning of a headache, there was almost immediate relief. Since then, I found that following protocol of taking one dropper every day for 30 days, even if there is no headache, helps to rid one of migraines. That is what worked for me. This is most blessed and welcome relief. I now keep a supply of Head Ease on hand.

—MAIRZIE

I love this formula! It works great, not just for sadness, but also for anxiety. I like to keep it on hand for the times that my hormones are going a bit crazy. My husband is a huge fan too. He likes the way it helps stabilize me. Well worth the money.

—MEREDITH

I took HB and T&C Formula for 1 month. I had my period last week with no cramps, and I didn't feel like kicking everything that got in my way, as that's how I feel on the week I get it. My husband usually knew when that time came. He would tiptoe around me that week, but this time I was my jolly self ALL month. Believe me; I didn't want to be like that. Thanks!

—MRS. GRAYBILL

I was suffering from Post Partum Depression, but HB Formula has given wonderful relief. I could cope so much better with stress and think clearer. Also, didn't experience such a weighed-down feeling.

—MRS. GINGERICH

I have taken the HB for a week and a half, three times a day. It got rid of my hot flashes! I am now taking it only once a day. Thank you!

—MRS. MAST

VISION

I was pleased with the results [of Eye-Can-C] for only being able to do it for 2 months. It was getting so it was hard to drive at night, but that has really changed. Thanks!

—J. WATSON

I have Glaucoma and am losing my sight. I feel the Eye-Can-See has stabilized my sight, and I am very pleased!

—ALAIRE

I have astigmatism, but in one eye it has improved! My prescription did not become any higher, which is a blessing.

—F. MILLER

I notice a major difference in 4 days. Night glare disappeared in 13 days by 90%. I rarely use my reading glasses. Three months later, eyesight has improved by 110%, and night glare is GONE.

—DR. STUART BLOCH (PATIENT ERIC M.)

ENDOMETRIOSIS, OVARIAN CYSTS

My pain started at twelve years old. An adult specialist finally told me I have endometriosis. During my two pregnancies, the pain lessened but always came back. I was ready to agree to the hysterectomy my doctor was recommending. I had gone two and a half years without a period. Then I found your catalog! I ordered the HB and T&C Formula right away and, after one week of taking it, I was pain-free and my menstrual cycle started! Today I would not be without your products; I have regular, pain-free cycles that only last five days, and I no longer have headaches. I can't believe I was so ready to spend thousands of dollars on surgery when your products are like $30.00 a bottle and work. Thank you so much for making available the herbs God provided to help others in need.

—Mrs. Waldner

I was taking the T&C for about a month after already having been doctored for endometriosis. They told me I had cysts all over my ovaries and that my tubes were completely clogged shut and that I would never be able to have children. This last time, I went in to have a checkup, and the doctor said my ovaries have cleared up a lot, and one of my tubes is beginning to be cleared out! I may have a chance at being pregnant after all! Thank you for such a great product!

—Missionary to Africa

About a year ago, I was looking at a hysterectomy; I have already had 3 D&Cs. My midwife gave me the T&C Formula, and I have not had to have a hysterectomy and feel great! I am using T&C as maintenance for approx 3 months once a year now.

—Mrs. Mast

The T&C is a great blessing to me. I had a cyst on my ovary the size of a baseball and was scheduled for surgery in 4 weeks. After using the T&C for 3 weeks, I went in for a checkup, and the cyst was gone!

—MRS. WEAVER

I am amazed at how well the T&C, HB Formula, and Progesterone Cream, used as you suggested, hve changed my life. No more painful and very long periods. My ovarian cyst has disappeared and my cycle is like clockwork! My doctor suggested surgery, but now that is no longer necessary. It has only been about 3 months, but what a difference! I feel like myself again! Thank you so much.

—HOLLY

MORNING SICKNESS

One of my clients was on an IV, too sick to keep down sips of water. Within 24 hours of taking the Stomach Aid, she quit vomiting and no longer needed the IV.

—MIDWIFE FROM VIRGINIA

Just wanted to let you know your product is the very first that has helped me so much. I feel like a new person and hardly realize I'm pregnant, something very unusual. I didn't know you could feel so good in such a short time after taking something for morning sickness that lasts all day long. I can work and exercise without getting sick! Thank you!

—MARTHA

I was pregnant with my first, and I was so sick I was in bed. I ordered some Morning Sickness Balm, and in a week's time I was feeling much better!

—MRS. HORST

This is my third pregnancy. I was sick for a week before I decided I am not going through feeling sick for three months. I looked around for help and got some herb teas to drink, but they were not much help. Then, my sister told me about Stomach Aid. She said to try it. I did and what a change! Now I can get up early in the morning to pack my husband's lunch and do my work. I am in my third month and have vomited only once!

—CAROLYN W

I was extremely sick 24 hours a day until I took the Stomach Aid I was extremely better within 24 hours of taking the formula!

—COLLEEN

I love your products. I took the Gentle Birth Formula, and I had a very easy labor. Now I'm expecting twins, and have been very sick. I tried Stomach Aid and was amazed at the results I got.

—MRS. WEAVER

I had good results with the Stomach Aid. I wouldn't be without it with another pregnancy. Thank you!

—MRS. FISHER

"Wonderful! It (Stomach Aid) consistently calmed my nausea, and I didn't have near the vomiting I did with my first 3 pregnancies."

—MRS. WEAVER

I still felt sick all night and vomited in the morning, but I didn't need to go back to the hospital for IV. Before I started taking it (Stomach Aid), I had been to the hospital 5 times.

—MRS. MILLER

Thanks for sending the Stomach Aid. It took a little over a week to get good results. I was kind of disappointed at first because nothing changed, but "BAM!" it all changed! I am still weak and can't work much, but 3 weeks without much food and water runs a body down quickly. Guess from now on, I'll have a bottle on hand so I can start using it as soon as I know I am pregnant. I have tried lots of different things in my 4 previous pregnancies, all to no avail. I appreciate your effort in making this product!

—MRS. MAST

My daughter was in bed and couldn't eat or drink. I gave her Stomach Aid and in 10 days, she was up and at work. She came for another bottle!

—SUSIE (MIDWIFE)

MISCARRIAGE AND HEAVY BLEEDING

Thank you so much for your good service. I was 2 months pregnant when I started with heavy bleeding. I used your C& B Formula and the bleeding completely stopped in 12 hours. Thank you so much for C&B Formula! I feel much better; I'd never want to be without C&B Formula the first few months of pregnancy! Thanks again for your wonderful service.

—MRS. MILLER

My favorite Mountain Meadow Herbs product is C&B Formula. Because is quickly helps when my uterus starts cramping and I start spotting in the first 3 months of pregnancy. Before I started using this, I had 2 miscarriages just a few months apart, and now since, I've had 5 healthy pregnancies. Thanks for a wonderful product

—ANN

Thanks for your C&B Formula. I was having a problem with spotting for two weeks already when I got your order and started taking the C&B Formula. The bleeding quit in two days. Thanks again!

—MRS. MILLER

I just want to tell you what great products you handle. I had one miscarriage and the second time I started bleeding again, so I looked through the MMH catalog. I saw the C&B Formula, so we got a 4 oz bottle. I took that for six hours and the bleeding completely stopped. I would never want to be without the C&B Formula during pregnancy. Thank you so much. God Bless You.

—MRS. YODER

I quit spotting after 2 days on the low dose of the C&B Formula. Thanks for sending it quickly! Now I have it on hand in case I start spotting again.

—RACHEL

VARICOSE VEINS

It really helps relieve my varicose veins. No more compression socks for me!

—BECKY

I am very thankful for Vari-Plex. My bulging veins are shrinking, and there is less soreness and itching as well.

—MRS. BYLER

I used your Gentle Birth formula for my last 2 babies! It worked! I normally went very late and instead was only 6-7 days late! And my labor was only 5 hours long instead of a day and a half!! I felt so much better afterwards, and my baby seemed more content too!! Also, I used Vari-Plex for my legs and they felt much better too!! Thanks for all your hard work. Glad God gave you the knowledge to mix what we need!!

—E. SAUDER

I am very well pleased with Vari-Plex. Within a week: minimal soreness, less swelling in my legs and feet, plus I bled very little after delivery!

—BERTHA

I am using Vascular Ease Lotion and Vari-Plex together with great results! Glad to find something that works! Mrs. Fisher I am just sold on this stuff! I'm pregnant right now and I wouldn't be without Vari-Plex. Send me more, please!

—MRS. STUTZMAN

When I was 2 months pregnant, I started taking your Vari-Plex and saw an improvement within a couple days. Thank you so much for your help!

—MRS. STOLTZFUS

I haven't found any other product that equals the results that "my ladies" get for their varicose vein problems, like Vari-Plex. Please send 10 more bottles, promptly. Thanks.

—MRS. GINGERICH (MIDWIFE)

PARASITES

My favorite product is Para-Rid, although I have seen positive benefits from using all of your products. We treated our whole family for parasites using Para-Rid and it worked. It was so easy to use for our large family, much easier than other methods, and the price is worth it. Consider how many future health problems you are avoiding! I believe parasites play a huge role in almost every health problem we have. Thank you for such helpful products!

—MICHELLE

I recommend all your products, but the one I have the best results with is the Para-Rid. I no longer hear my children and husband grind their teeth and talk in their sleep.

—F. BORNTAGER

Our daughter has suffered health problems for many years, including anxiety and depression. She is on the last day of taking Para-Rid. We can't believe how many movements of parasites she has passed! We are looking for better days for her!

—MRS.KAUFMAN

My daughter always craved sweets until I used the Para-Rid. Now all she wants is fruits & veggies. Thank you!

—C. HERRON

The Para-Rid is a good product. My child is finally gaining weight!

—N. YODER

I used the Para-Rid for my little boy who didn't like to eat anything besides sweets. [I am] very glad he enjoys good food now and sleeps through the night. Also, is friskier!

—LYDIA

We were very pleased with the results of using Para-Rid. That is why we are ordering some again.

—S. HABEGGER

The kids started eating a lot better and our 3-year-old was a lot calmer.

—EMMA

I just want to say thank you, thank you, thank you. I'm so happy and impressed with the results of Para-Rid. My 5-year-old daughter did not want to eat anything. It was so frustrating for me to see how other kids ate everything and she was so selective. On the second day of treatment she began to ask me for more and more food, she had never wanted to try chicken soup and this time she took it all and ate all the vegetables! She ate fruit, and she tried new food that she had never wanted to try before. Her sleep habits also changed: She went to bed early and woke early too, with lots of energy but without dark circles around her eyes. What a change! She was a girl with many gases, but after 6 days of taking the Para-Rid she doesn't have any more digestive problems, and in a week she gained 2 pounds. All the family had a great week. Now we are waiting for the next full moon to give her the next treatment.

—KAROL

CLEANSING

I find myself taking the stairs now and attacking my work with renewed vigor. I love this stuff!

—B. W. ARIZONA

INFERTILITY

I wanted to let you know I am finally expecting our first child, before finishing the three month supply of Whole Body/Colon Cleanse I ordered and the Para-Rid! We have been praying and trying to conceive for twelve years!

—ANNIE

We have been married 7 years and were unable to conceive, but then we did the liver and the gall bladder cleanses and conceived a month after the treatment.

—CAROLINA

After a month of Lega-C herbs and Fruitful Vine, I conceived. I am expecting my first child by Mother's Day! I am so thankful and feel blessed to have found you.

—ANONYMOUS

I wasn't half way through my first bottle (Fruitful Vine) until I had a positive test. How excited and thankful we are.

—MRS. MAST

Five years after our youngest son was born, my husband and I wanted to have another baby, but I was unable to conceive. After hearing a friend's testimony on the Fruitful Vine, we decided to give it a try although we hardly dared hope it would work for us. It arrived while I was having my period so I went on it right away taking almost twice the recommended dose thinking either this stuff is going to work, or not! Two weeks later we were in shock when we read a positive pregnancy test!! It must absolutely be the best infertility product available, thank you.

—RUTHANN

I've had trouble conceiving, so my midwife suggested the Fruitful Vine. I took it for one month; then the next month I got pregnant. I also took the Vitamin C. Thanks to the makers of the Fruitful Vine!

—MRS. BEILER

I have been taking the Fruitful Vine forever, (10months) and just got a positive test! I doubled my dose after talking with a friend. IT WORKED!

—MARY KATHERINE

I'm very, very well pleased by your supplements. I took the Fruitful Vine with Vitamin C for 7 weeks and it worked. We now have an 18 month old daughter who is so healthy and happy. I was so thankful for the Maxi-Milk, because my milk supply was low, and I wanted to keep on nursing. So I took that, and within days I had plenty of milk. Thank you and God Bless You!

—E.C.

I started the Lega-C-Herbs 3 months ago. My sperm count was 7 million and now it is at 30 million. Something is working!

—J. PEACHY

After being married almost 7 years, and after one month on Lega-C-Herbs for me and one month of Fruitful Vine and Vitamin C for my wife, we were expecting! Thank you for your products and God Bless you all.

—ANONYMOUS

Your products for men have helped me. Thank you! I have used them for a few months and have best results when I also take them and the vitamins regularly. Something has been helping as we are expecting our first child. My impotence is better.

—OHIO

After conceiving our first child easily and naturally, we were disappointed when we were not getting pregnant again after several years of trying for a second child. During the 5 years of trying, we saw OBGYN, Fertility, and Naturopathic doctors and did many tests. My husband's sperm count was good, and motility was good. However, the morphology was abnormal so sperm could not penetrate the egg. Doctors said the only way we could get pregnant was through IVF. We decided to try natural healing. We added more plant-based protein to my husband's diet, adjusted some lifestyle habits, and took both Lega-C Herbs, and ProGentor. After 3 months he was tested again and is completely back to normal! We are so hopeful that we will conceive naturally. I am convinced that both of the products have helped the numbers to move, and to move as quickly as they have.

—ANONYMOUS

ADD, BEDWETTING, STUTTERING

A friend gave her son, who is school aged, Herbal Calcium and she noticed he had not had any bed-wetting. Before, he would wet the bed every now and then. She quit giving him the formula, and he had a couple accidents. Started him on the formula again, and bed wetting stopped. This is the only thing the mother did differently. He was noticed as being more alert in school too. Not sure what dosage she gave him.

—ANONYMOUS

I use Herbal Calcium for our 4-year-old and 1-year-old. Without it, they seem to be all over the place and don't have much focus. Even our baby sitter has noticed when we've forgotten to give it to them. Our 7-year-old uses Natural Attention-Aid, and it seems to help her focus better with her schoolwork.

—MRS. RIEHL

My nonverbal son (diagnosed with autism) has had much better focus and self-control since starting this; also, he is sleeping better and is less aggressive. If we miss a day of taking this everyone in the house knows it. He must notice a difference because he asks for it every day. It's made huge improvements in his behavior, and I am so thankful. This is an answer to prayer. Thank you!!!

—TARA

Works wonders on teething babies and calming children. We have a set of identical twin boys who have extreme (high maintenance) natures. More than once, I have reached for liquid calcium, and it calms them right down. It helps them be able to focus for schoolwork too.

—HANNAH

I used your herb for ADD for our son, and we could really tell a difference. He did better in school. His teacher asked him, "Is Mom giving you magic medicine?" It made us feel good. Also, his bedwetting stopped. I LOVE your products!

—MRS. SCHWARTZ

My son who is in 5th grade was taking the herbs for ADD, but we ran out at the end of the year. After about two weeks, we could really tell the difference. When at school, he is able to focus and concentrate; otherwise he fiddles.

—AMOS M

After a friend's suggestion, we tried Natural Attention Aid and Herbal Calcium for our 4-year-old son. After 6 months of regular use, we stopped using it for 10 days to make sure he really needed it. During those 10 days he started bedwetting, had night tremors, his speech became very bad with a lot of stuttering, and he became very unmanageable and unkind. When we put him back on the Natural Attention Aid and Herbal Calcium, everything disappeared, and he now behaves as a normal child.

—MRS. BYLER

Natural Attention Aid has helped for concentration at work for me, a 21-year-old. I wish I would have started it at a younger age. Thank you!
—STOLTZFUS

For years I was searching for help for our ADD children. Some products helped a little. I decided to try your Natural Attention Aid. The results are amazing. We don't want to be without.

—MRS. ZOOK

My son can cope better with everyday activities and isn't so grouchy anymore! Thanks!

—MARIA

Our sons, age twelve and nineteen, are really pleased with this product for their bed- wetting problem! It really works! After all these years we've finally found something that works. God Bless and keep you!

—SADIE K

Our son (in first grade) had poor grades, and it was difficult for him to concentrate on his lessons. After the first bottle of Natural Attention Aid, we could tell how much it helped him. It also stopped his bedwetting problem.

—MRS. SCHWARTZ

COLDS, FLU, AND ASTHMA

The Herbal Calcium keeps you from getting weak if you have a high fever.

—EDNA

I don't know what I would do without you guys! Our son has half a heart, and as long as we use the Herbal Respiratory and Infant Immune-Booster, he stays healthier than our other boys with no difficulties. Thank you so much for making such wonderful products.

—D. WEAVER

TESTIMONIES

I really like the Herbal Respiratory. As soon as the little ones start with a cold, I give it to them, and they get over it much sooner. Thank you for great products!

—L. YODER

I haven't found anything that works half as well as the Infant Immune Booster, for our whole family.

—DANIEL Y.

We've used your Herbal Respiratory and Infant Immune Booster more than any other product you have. We don't like to be without it. We like it if we think we're getting sick or have a cold or sore throat, and I like it because it's okay to take if you're expecting or nursing.

—M. GIROD

I think your Herbal Respiratory and Infant Immune Boost are just wonderful! I usually get laryngitis and bad colds and have to go to the doctor to get antibiotics. But this year, I took your Infant Immune Boost and Herbal Respiratory and did not have to go see the doctor! I could actually speak, and I like that I could take it while nursing my baby. I also gave the herbs to him with excellent results!

—MULLET

I don't want to be without Infant Immune Boost. If our 13-month-old starts with a cold, I start her on Infant Immune Boost. Almost always clears it up in a couple of days!

—YODER

I really like Herbal Respiratory for our whole family. One winter, we had three cases of pneumonia, so the next winter, we used lots of Herbal Respiratory, and we didn't have a single visit to the doctor. It also prevents our children from getting croup. I do not want to be without!

—WITMER

The Herbal Respiratory DOES WORK. I have been using it on all my children, ages 16 months, 3 years, and 4 years. I give them 1/8 tsp four times a day for approx. 7 days during a cold or if exposed to a cold. Sometimes, I use it along with an Echinacea tincture. WOW! Hardly any coughing, and the croup just dried up!

—ANONYMOUS)

I am sending you a testimonial about Herbal Respiratory. Lung support seems to be our main need in our house, because we have two with asthma and one that gets croup very easy. I find that if I start out and give Herbal Respiratory 4 times a day to my children WITH an immune boosting formula like Infant Immune Boost (or something similar), the cold just disappears within days. I like to give it for about 7-10 days. No more doctor visits or emergency room runs when I use this. I am saving up so I can get 6 bottles at a time. If they are having trouble breathing, I give an extra dose. My daughter's croup was better within a day or so. I just can't find another product that is so easy to administer, works so well, and can be used from a tiny infant to adult and even nursing mothers. If I ever have another baby, I plan to have this on hand. My second daughter had RSV when she was a month old. If only I would have had Herbal Respiratory and Infant Immune Boost she probably would have never had to go to the doctor or hospital at all! Thanks for making a great product! God Bless!

—AMANDA W

I use the Herbal Respiratory for my 3 children a lot. When I treat them for a cold, I start with an immune boosting formula and add Herbal Respiratory for a minimum of 10 days. The colds and coughs disappear! I plan to keep purchasing this from you!

—MRS. WITMER

I have a two-year-old daughter with Down Syndrome. She seems to have a weakness fighting colds, flu's, and respiratory issues. Herbal Respiratory has been a great blessing to us. We've had a good winter. Although she had upper respiratory congestion most of the winter, Herbal Respiratory and God's grace have kept her from getting sick!

—MRS. HORST

With Herbal Respiratory, we were able to quit using aerosol treatments for our son with asthma!

—BARBARA M

I love your products. Our 6-month baby had a bad cough and mucus. The Infant Immune Boost and Herbal Respiratory really helped with the fever too. Thank you so much.

—SUSAN

This tincture (Herbal Respiratory) has been a real help to us this winter! My husband has been having respiratory problems ever since we came to Indiana last January. After recurrent colds, he started taking the Herbal Respiratory each time his symptoms began, and most times, his cold did not advance further. Thanks so much!!

—EILEEN W

STRESS AND NERVOUSNESS

I used 2 doses of your Stress and Sleep last evening, and I slept better than I have for a long time. Please send me two 4 oz bottles. Thanks again for your prompt service.

—ROBERT TROYER

Since I started using Stress and Sleep, I have been able to stop using my prescription medication to help me sleep for the first time in 16 years.

—MRS. ZOOK

I have had a tight stomach for a long time. My chiropractor said my transverse colon is sluggish, but nothing seemed to help until I started with the Stress and Sleep. In a few days my tightness was gone. Thanks for a good product!

—BARBARA

My husband uses Stress and Sleep and has definitely noticed a difference in the quality of his rest. We're both under a lot of stress, and I'm glad to have found something that helps.

—MRS. HOCHSTETLER

Stress and Sleep relaxes me!

—MRS. YODER

FATIGUE AND INSOMNIA

I like the Herbal Calcium. I give it to my 1-year-old and 2-year-old at bedtime. They sleep so much better. I don't want to be without it.

—GLENDA

I suffer from chronic fatigue, which causes me to have a great deal of muscle/joint aches. I had been taking a calcium/magnesium supplement, but the amount my body required resulted in a laxative effect with the pains recurring shortly after taking. Due to sensitivities, I had to get the Herbal Calcium custom made blend, which removed the offending herbs. Since taking this herbal treasure, my pains have diminished greatly. I love that I can take it multiple times a day if needed without a laxative effect, but a calming, tension-relieving effect for my skeleton system. Our kids take it at night to help relax them and give them more restful sleep and combat growing pains. We love this stuff.

—T. ADAMS

I am sleeping better. I am taking BedTime Drops, Herbal Calcium, and Stress and Sleep. I feel way more refreshed. I am no longer taking naps.

—MIRIAM

Since my last pregnancy three years ago, I have had problems with sleeping. I would lie in bed sometimes 1-2 hours before falling asleep and be up at least 2-3 times in the night, sometimes more. After taking the Herbal Calcium, I drop off almost as soon as my head touches the pillow and only get up once during the night. I love it and wouldn't want to be without it!

—TENA

Thank you for the BedTime Drops. I have brain and liver cancer; these herbs are the only thing that makes sleep possible for me.

—OHIO

I love these drops! I'm nearing 40 years old and have started to wake up almost nightly around 4 a.m. I toss and turn for the next couple of hours, and right when I should be waking up, I'm finally starting to fall back asleep. So frustrating! These drops have changed all that. I'm getting a full night's sleep and I feel great in the morning. My husband and my son adore them as well. Good stuff!

—KATIE W.

After years of waking at odd times throughout the night unable to resume sleep and feeling groggy during the day, I am amazed at how this small amount of liquid heaven helps me fall asleep, keeps my mind from racing, and allows me to sleep fully through the night. I awake feeling more refreshed and energized. Best sleep aid I have used, and I have used many.

—TMICE

ADRENALS

I love Adren-L-Aid. I feel it has helped me a lot. I used to get panic attacks, which I now believe was adrenal exhaustion. I thank God for a good product like this one, and I thank you for explaining in detail what the product is for, or I'd probably never have realized I need it.

—MRS. BYLER

My favorite product is the Adren-L-Aid because it helps give me energy and it reduces stress. If only more doctors knew about this, it could help so many more people! Thank you so much!

—DAVID R.

I don't handle stress well and have suffered from anxiety and fatigue in the past. I used to be a zombie without my coffee, too. As a mom of two small kids and a newborn, I worry about getting through the day in one piece. I was shocked that on the first day of taking Adren-L-Aid, I required NO coffee and had enough steam to make it till my husband got home from work. I was able to clean, make dinner, AND keep my temper with the kids. I am thoroughly impressed with and grateful for this product and want my husband to start taking it!

—ERIN BUSSIAN

Thank you for your great formulas! My husband started taking the Adren-L-Aid and was able to stop using tobacco after 15 years with very little withdrawal! It has truly been a blessing!

—MRS. COBLENTZ

I love Adren-L-Aid. I feel it has helped me a lot. I used to get panic attacks, which I believe was adrenal exhaustion. I thank God for a good product like that, and I thank you for explaining in detail what the product is for or I'd probably never have realized I need it.

—MRS. BYLER

I'm very pleased with your Adren-L-Aid II. I have more energy and am able to get a good night's sleep without my medication.

—MRS. PETERSHEIM

By taking 1/2 a bottle (Adren-L-Aid), our son has lost 15 lbs, and he is able to do things he couldn't do before! It's totally amazing! For a whole week, he was varnishing and he didn't have any chest pains or headaches!

—JOHN D

I can work a full day and still feel good instead of weary, tired and blue. Thank you for a wonderful product.

—SHARON M.

For years I have suffered from adrenal exhaustion. Bovine supplementation and other adrenal aids were insufficient in restoring my energy, sleep issues, and other adrenal- related issues. After just two days of using Adren-L-Aid I began to feel like the person I remembered before adrenal exhaustion. My energy, mood and sleep patterns are stable, and the herbs are not overly stimulating like others I have tried. Wish I had known about this company's brand at the onset of my adrenal issues.

—TMICE

ANTI-SPASMODIC

Our son has made a dramatic change since being on your Anti-Spasmodic tincture. He tried another brand, but he went into convulsions, like my dad used to. Needless to say, we are ALL well pleased and happy to have our "Sunshine" boy back to his normal self. We don't want to run out. We truly appreciate being able to find something to help him. Thanks again and God Bless!

—L. SCHROCK

This is more effective than my prescription. It doesn't make me drowsy or angry like my prescription does. I'm very pleased with this product. Thank you for this. I never go without it.

—ANONYMOUS

SHOULDER PAIN

I have suffered from shoulder pain for years. After seeing a naturopath I realized my liver needed help. After two weeks of regularly taking the LiverGlow the pain is completely gone and my digestion is much improved.

—MRS. BYLER

YEAST INFECTION

I have had problems with yeast for over twenty years and have never been able to take anything for it because I would be allergic to the product, or it didn't agree with my system. The Yeast X package is the first product that I have found that I am able to use, and it is working great after only a month. I want to order more to complete the three months.

—M KELLY

Your Yeast X Package is giving me very positive results. It's the first product that works after years of trying to doctor my yeast. Thanks, my nails are slowly coming back to normal. Your products are very good.

—MRS. SCHWARTZ

I'm getting good results with the Yeast X and hope to do the Adren-L-Aid in a few months. As long as Mountain Meadow Herbs exists, you'll find me as one of your satisfied and happy customers.

—LINDA

WEIGHT LOSS

I took Adren-L-Aid and LiverGlow along with Herbal Calcium. I lost 40 pounds in a couple months. I was more energetic and more active.

—S. HAMM

In spite of daily exercise, dieting and trying a lot of different supplements, my ideal weight stayed out of reach. My husband brought me a sample of Weight Control, and six weeks later I had lost an astonishing thirty pounds just in time for our daughter's wedding!

—MRS. MILLER

I notice my appetite has decreased and it takes less for me to feel full since I'm taking the Weight Control.

—JORAM

I have lost 15 pounds and two dress sizes since I started Weight Control. I exercised when possible, but the biggest difference was a big change in how much it takes to satisfy me, and I am also not hungry all the time. I lost the weight six months ago, and I have not regained any of it.

—GARBER

CUSTOMER COMMENTS

I wanted to thank you all for being so helpful with my shipment and going the extra mile to make things work for me. I have never had customer service that was so prompt and helpful! It has been a pleasure to work with you and I am sure I will be working more with you in the future.

—KRISTINA L

In July of 2005, I had cellulites in my leg, and I asked you for something to help clear it up. I had a prescription from the doctor, but it did not clear it up. You did research on it and gave me Gotu Kola: one bottle to put on my leg and one to take internally. After several bottles, it cleared up! Just wanted to let you know what the results were. Thank you for taking time and interest in my case and thanks goes to the giver of these wonderful herbs!

—MRS. STUTZMAN

Just wanted to take a minute to let you know how much we appreciate your product. What a find! To be able to purchase excellent quality (tinctures) liquid herbs. We took one of your products with us to the chiropractor to be muscle-tested, and we're very pleased that it proved to test clean of any pesticide residue or any other environmental toxins that would be harmful to the body, which seems to be harder to accomplish these days. Thanks again and May God Bless your work. I can't wait to try other products.

—LINDSAY R

REAL STORIES FROM REAL PEOPLE

These are a sample of testimonies from real people who shared with us their experiences in using the herbal remedies we carefully created. The products are available from Mountain Meadow Herbs, and they are extracted and formulated using the same process I developed in my home ten years ago. Calls are still answered by a team member trained in compassion and caring because all employees remained with the company after its sale.

The FDA has not approved the information contained in this guide. While it is based on the wisdom passed down through generations and that has, in many cases, been validated by modern science, it is not intended to replace a physician's care or advice, or to treat, prevent, or cure any disease. Freedom comes with responsibility; please do not choose herbal remedies or dietary supplements if you are unwilling to also assume the risk. The author is not responsible for the outcome of the choices of the reader. This information is provided both to assist those who are interested in natural solutions in making wise decisions and to add to the growing awareness of the value and hope that can be found in herbal remedies and dietary supplements.

HYPERHEALTH SOFTWARE
info@hyperhealth.com
886-811-4921
www.hyperhealth.com

NUTRITIONAL HERBOLOGY
Written by Mark Pederson
The Bulk Herb Store
26W 6th Ave. | Lobelville, TN 37091
877-278-4257
www.thebulkherbstore.com

THE CURE FOR ALL DISEASES
Written by Hulda Regehr Clark, Ph.D., N.D.
Mountain Meadow Herbs
P.O. Box 9227 | Kalispell, MT 59904
888-528-8615
www.mountainmeadowherbs.com

MOMMY DIAGNOSTICS
Written By Shonda Parker
Naturally Healthy
P.O.Box 360 | Calhoun, LA 71225
www.naturallyhealthy.org

TAKING CHARGE OF YOUR FERTILITY
Written by Toni Weschler, MPH
Mountain Meadow Herbs
P.O. Box 9227 | Kalispell, MT 59904
888-528-8615
www.mountainmeadowherbs.com

To locate a store near you where herbal products formulated by
Kathy can be purchased please visit
www.savingtristan.com (store locator).

For additional copies of this book:

MOMS HERB GUIDE
P.O. Box 9380
Kalispell, MT 59904
406-756-6654
www.savingtristan.com

THE WILLIAM AND LYDIA FOUNDATION
P.O. Box 9380
Kalispell, MT 59904
406-212-2255
Email: info@thewilliamandlydiafoundation.com

APPENDIX

V

Varicose Veins 34-35

Vari-Plex 34

Vascular Ease Lotion 35

Vision Loss 70, 72

Vitamin C 23, 42-43, 59, 74

W

Weight control 96

Weight loss 47, 93, 96-97

Whole Body Colon Cleanse 39-40, 44-46

Y

Yeast die off 40

Yeast infection 39-40, 44-45, 47, 49-51

Yeast X 40